HEALTH AND FITNESS THROUGH PHYSICAL ACTIVITY

AMERICAN COLLEGE OF SPORTS MEDICINE SERIES

SKI CONDITIONING

Merle Foss and James G. Garrick

**CONDITIONING FOR DISTANCE RUNNING:
THE SCIENTIFIC ASPECTS**

Jack Daniels, Robert Fitts, and George Sheehan

THE PHYSIOLOGY AND BIOMECHANICS OF CYCLING

Irvin Faria and Peter Cavanaugh

**HEALTH AND FITNESS THROUGH
PHYSICAL ACTIVITY**

Michael Pollock, Jack Wilmore, and Samuel Fox

HEALTH AND FITNESS THROUGH PHYSICAL ACTIVITY

MICHAEL L. POLLOCK
Director, Cardiac Rehabilitation Program and
Human Performance Laboratory
Department of Medicine
Mount Sinai Medical Center
Milwaukee, Wisconsin
And Former
Director of Research
Institute for Aerobics Research
Dallas, Texas

JACK H. WILMORE
Head, Department of Physical Education
University of Arizona
Tucson, Arizona

SAMUEL M. FOX III
Professor of Medicine
Director, Cardiology Exercise Laboratory
Georgetown University Medical Center
Washington, D.C.

JOHN WILEY & SONS

New York   Santa Barbara   Chichester   Brisband   Toronto

Copyright © 1978, by John Wiley & Sons, Inc.

All rights reserved. Published simultaneously in Canada.

No part of this book may be reproduced by any means, nor
transmitted, nor translated into a machine language without the written permission of the publisher.

Library of Congress Cataloging in Publication Data
Pollock, Michael L
  Health and fitness through physical activity.

  (College of Sports Medicine series)
  Includes bibliographies and index.
  1. Exercise. 2. Physical fitness. I. Wilmore,
Jack H., 1938-   joint author. II. Fox, Samuel
Mickle, 1923-   joint author. III. Title.
IV. Series: American College of Sports Medicine.
College of Sports Medicine series.
RA781. P59   613.7'1   78-495
ISBN 0-471-69285-9

Printed in the United States of America

10 9 8 7 6 5 4 3 2 1

DEDICATION

This book is dedicated to our patient, understanding, and lovely wives:
JUDY, DOTTIE, AND MARY ALICE

FOREWORD

During the past 10 years, a tremendous explosion of knowledge has occured in the exercise and sport sciences. New theories in the coaching and training of athletes have emerged, technological breakthroughs have allowed a better understanding of how people perform and adapt to the stress of exercise, and we now have a better understanding as to how exercise can improve both the quality and quantity of life. In addition, the population of the United States has become more conscious of physical fitness and has started exercising on their own, with little or no knowledge of what to do, or how to go about it. Consequently, many commercial enterprises have resolved to satisfy this basic consumer need. Although many of these enterprises have provided valuable consumer services, there are many others that have not had the consumer's best interests at heart and have taken advantage of the general lack of knowledge of the average consumer.

In 1973, the American College of Sports Medicine, at the suggestion of their former President, Dr. Howard G. Knuttgen, planned a series of volumes to help bridge the widening gap between the latest research in the exercise and sport sciences and the consumer. The purpose of this Series was to bring to the level of the average consumer, the facts and basic information related to exercise in general, and individual sports specifically, in an interesting and unbiased manner. Dr. David L. Costill, currently President of the American College of Sports Medicine, was asked to initiate this Series.

The American College of Sports Medicine's Series is an exciting step forward in the area of consumer education. Each volume is co-authored by authorities in their respective areas, who were selected for their ability to communicate their ideas at a very practical and fundamental level. While each of these authors is a recognized scientist, each volume represents an attempt to apply the teachings and findings of science to the better understanding of and participation in various activities and sports. It is the intent of this Series to develop a more informed consumer and to stimulate widespread participation in a variety of activities and sports.

JACK H. WILMORE
Chairperson, Publications Committee
American College of Sports Medicine

About the Authors

Michael L. Pollock is an exercise physiologist who is Director of Cardiac Rehabilitation at the Center for the Evaluation of Human Performance, Mount Sinai Medical Center, Milwaukee, Wisconsin. He also holds academic appointments as an Associate Professor, Department of Medicine, University of Wisconsin Medical School, Madison; and Clinical Professor, Department of Health and Physical Education, University of Wisconsin, Milwaukee. He was graduated from the University of Arizona and received his M.S. and Ph.D. from the University of Illinois, Champaign. Dr. Pollock was formerly Director of the Adult Fitness Program, Wake Forest University, Winston-Salem, N.C., and most recently Director of Research, Institute for Aerobics Research, Dallas, Texas. He has consulted with the Dallas Cowboys and Dallas Tornado professional teams, and Olympic distance runners.

Jack H. Wilmore is an exercise physiologist who is Professor and Head of the Department of Physical Education, University of Arizona, Tucson. He was graduated from the University of California, Santa Barbara, where he also received his M.S. His Ph.D. was received from the University of Oregon. Dr. Wilmore was formerly coordinator of the Adult Fitness Program at the University of California, Davis, and most recently Executive Director of the National Athletic Health Institute, Los Angeles, California. He has consulted with many athletic teams, such as the Oakland Raiders, San Francisco 49ers, and Los Angeles Rams and Dodgers, and is currently President of the American College of Sports Medicine.

Samuel M. Fox is a cardiologist who is Professor of Medicine and Director of the Cardiology Exercise Program, Georgetown University Medical Center, Washington, D.C. He was graduated from the University of Pennsylvania School of Medicine. Dr. Fox was formerly Assistant Director, National Heart and Lung Institute, National Institutes of Health; and Chief, Heart Disease and Stroke Control Program, U.S. Public Health Serice. He is a past President of the American College of Cardiology and past Vice-President of the American College of Sports Medicine. Dr. Fox is a charter member of the President's Council on Physical Fitness and Sports and was chairman of the Exercise Committee of the American Heart Association.

PREFACE

The authors have been involved in all aspects of physical fitness work and during the past fifteen years have published many research papers dealing with exercise and physical fitness. This book is an attempt to synthesize this work, as well as other information concerning health and fitness, into a compact, concise, and easily read volume.

The authors wanted to go beyond the idea of purely describing facts, but more importantly, explain to the readers why certain procedures are followed in evaluating fitness and prescribing exercise. Thus, it is hoped that this text will give the future participant and long-time exercise enthusiast better insight into many aspects of health and physical fitness.

The book is divided into seven subtopics with Section 1 giving a general overview of the need for exercise and fitness and how it is an integral part of preventive medicine program. Section 2 attempts to take the research findings on exercise, health maintenance, and performance and translate them into logical, down-to-earth terms. Readers who are not interested in the scientific basis of exercise and fitness should omit Section 2 and go directly to Section 3. Section 3 outlines and describes the various aspects of medical screening and fitness evaluation procedures. This section mentions several categories of tests which have different levels of sophistication and cost. More detailed information concerning testing protocols and how to administer tests are described in Appendix A. Section 4 explains exercise prescription and emphasizes the individualized approach; that is, exercise is prescribed individually depending upon the participants, level of fitness and health status, goals, and interests. Section 5 deals with rehabilitation of the cardiac patient, Section 6, nutritional aspects, of human performance, and Section 7, special considerations for exercise programs. Section 7 takes into consideration important aspects; such as shoes and clothing to use when beginning your exercise program; the importance of warming up and cooling down; special considerations for heat, cold, altitude and air pollution; age and sex considerations; motivation for short and long term exercise programs; and special exercise programs that can be used at home or while traveling.

The preparation of this book was exciting and challenging for the authors and hopefully it will meet its designated purpose. Such a challenge and fulfillment is never a result of a few individuals, but includes many persons and organizations. The initial stimulus for this manuscript came from the Publications Committee of the American College of Sports Medicine, Dr. David Costill, chairman. Appreciation goes to Mrs. Mona Pickens, who typed the entire manuscript with remarkable speed and accuracy and with tremendous dedication; and, to Ms. Holly Hausmann who helped in the typing of the first draft of a couple sections. Appreciation also goes to Mrs. Mary Faye Marks who helped proof and edit the final manuscript. A very special appreciation goes to Dr. Larry Gettman, John Ayres, and Ann Ward who gave advice and made special contributions to various segments of this book. And lastly, appreciation goes to Thomas K. Cureton, Ph.D., professor emeritus and Director of the Adult Fitness Research Laboratory, University of Illinois, from 1941 to 1967; Albert R. Behnke, M.D., pioneer in sports medicine research; and W. Proctor Harvey, M.D., Director, Division of Cardiology, Georgetown University Medical Center, for their inspiration, strong leadership, and influence on our lives and thus, helped make this book possible.

MICHAEL L. POLLOCK

JACK H. WILMORE

SAMUEL M. FOX, III

January, 1978

CONTENTS

HEALTH AND FITNESS THROUGH PHYSICAL ACTIVITY

Section 1

Physical Activity, Health and Designed Exercise Programs: An Overview

INTRODUCTION

Since the dawn of the Industrial Revolution, technology has advanced at an astounding rate. During this time, we have seen the transformation of a basically hard-working, physically active, rural-based society into a population of anxious and troubled city dwellers and suburbanites, who may get faint of heart at the very thought of exercise and vigorous physical activity. Advances in modern technology have enabled our present-day society to exist in a world where the concept of hard or even moderate physical work is as obsolete and unfashionable as outhouses and running boards on automobiles. Hand or push lawn mowers have been replaced by power lawn mowers, which, in turn, have been replaced by artificial turf. Elevators and escalators have replaced stairs—just try to find an open stairway in a modern high rise! The walk to the corner market has been replaced by a short drive to the supermarket in the neighborhood shopping center. Frequently, the time spent driving to the shopping center is less than the time spent circling the parking lot in hopes of getting one of the prime parking spaces directly in front of the store. We are constantly looking for ways to make life even easier—easier, that is, from the viewpoint of conserving effort and human energy. What do we do with all of this effort and energy that we have *saved*? The question might be better phrased, what does a sedentary life-style do to us as individuals? Do we profit or do we suffer?

If you have ever taken the time or had the interest in studying the human body and how it works, that is, human anatomy and physiology, you cannot help but be impressed with the intricate manner in which the body functions, and the delicate manner in which the body systems are so consistently in perfect harmony. Disrupt that harmony in even a very simple way, for example, the common cold or the morning hangover, and the whole body suffers. There is a growing area of knowledge that is beginning to demonstrate without question that physical inactivity and the increased sedentary nature of our daily living habits are a serious threat to the body, causing major deterioration in normal body function. Such common and serious medical problems as coronary heart disease, hypertension, obesity, anxiety and depression, and lower back problems have been either directly or indirectly associated with our lack of physical activity. Each of these will be discussed briefly and their link to physical inactivity will be established.

In addition to physical inactivity, a number of additional factors are associated with the above diseases or medical problems, including smoking, overeating, improper diet, excessive alcohol consumption, and emotional stress. These are all complications of our modern life-style. To make the most significant impact on improving general health and avoiding disease and disability, it is important to make a major change in life-style. To start an exercise program but continue a two pack-a-day cigarette habit greatly limits the gains that can be made from such an activity program. As a result of the nearly complete conquest of the usual infectious diseases, a change in life-style is at present the very essence of preventive medicine. It is important that such changes should be adopted or initiated as early in life as possible. Frequently, making the commitment to start an exercise program is the key to making a whole series of changes in daily living, breaking habits that have been longstanding.

In subsequent sections it will be explained how the person who exercises frequently and with at least moderate vigor for more than a few minutes each day will have some predictable increase in his or her capacity to tolerate this effort with relative ease. Because of the heavy personal discomfort and disability associated with disease, as well as the costs, it is of more than academic interest to know if there is a preventive effect that can be stimulated by a physical activity program acceptably modest in its demands. This is discussed in connection with various diseases that present some, but clearly not all, of today's major medical problems.

ANXIETY AND DEPRESSION. Anxiety and depression are two undesirable psychological states that have reached pandemic proportions over the past decade. Emotional disturbance may be the cause of more marital, professional, and social distress than many organic diseases combined. Anxiety can be defined as a vague feeling of nervousness, apprehension, and uncertainty, and is similar to the feeling associated with fear. But with anxiety, the feeling is usually not associated with a specific cause or threat. It can produce confusion and distorted perceptions of time and space, and of motivations and the meaning of events. It can interfere with learning and normal functioning by lowering concentration, impairing memory, and decreasing the ability to relate one item to another. Depression is characterized by a sense of hopelessness, self-depreciation, bitterness, regret, and a slowing of emotional processes as well as mental and body functioning. It has been reported that over 50 percent of all patients hospitalized with emotional illness have been diagnosed as suffering from various depressive disorders. Ten million Americans are reported to suffer from anxiety neurosis.

The role of exercise in preventing and treating individuals who are anxious and depressed has been the focus of considerable research over the past few years. Dr. William P. Morgan, a sport psychologist, has summarized this research in a recent book and has made the following generalizations. Individuals who participate in a vigorous exercise program consistently report that they "feel better" as a result of the vigorous exercise. This sensation of "feeling better" appears to represent an alteration in tension and anxiety. Anxiety levels are reduced following vigorous exercise in both normal men and women, as well as anxious neurotics. Finally, there does appear to be a reduction in levels of depression following chronic physical activity. Morgan concludes by stating that acute and chronic physical activity of a vigorous nature offers a unique and effective method of reducing anxiety and depression.

"TYPE A" BEHAVIOR PATTERN. Dr. David Jenkins, a psychologist from Boston, describes a behavior pattern ("Type A") that is associated with the development of coronary heart disease. He states that the overt behavioral syndrome or style of living is characterized by extremes of competitiveness, striving for achievement, agressiveness (sometimes stringently repressed), haste, impatience, restlessness, hyperalertness, explosiveness of speech, tenseness of facial musculature, and feelings of being under the pressure of time and under the challenge of responsibility. The Type A behavioral pattern has also been associated with many of the other fisk factors, such as elevated serum cholesterol and triglycerides, elevated blood pressure, and cigarette smoking. In order to help combat the heart disease problem, many researchers recommend that emphasis be placed on behavior modification.

MUSCULOSKELETAL DISEASE OR DISABILITY. Although not resulting from the most sophisticated, controlled experimental study, there is good reason to believe that skiers, tennis players, and other seasonal sport participants who are otherwise physically active have a lower rate of injury and discomfort than their sedentary colleagues when they take up these activities upon return of the season. There is also good evidence that those who remain active in their later years retain greater bone, ligament, and tendon strength, and thus are less prone to fractures and tears.

LOWER BACK PROBLEMS. Lower back problems are found in a very high percentage of our adult population. It has been documented that 80 percent of back pain is due to musculoskeletal deficiencies, stress, and tension. It has been accepted for some time that poor posture and muscle weakness are the major cause of most back complaints. In one study of several hundred adults who had chronic complaints of lower back problems, almost 80 percent of these patients had muscle weakness and stiffness diagnosed as the cause, and only 20 percent were the result of a specific disease, lesion, or anatomical anomaly. The patients who were diagnosed as having muscular weakness were treated through a therapeutic exercise program that emphasized development of strength and flexibility. Of the total population under study, 233 cases were followed for approximately eight years. The symptoms of these patients improved with improved strength and flexibility. Eighty-two percent reported success with the program two to eight years following the treatment. Thus, exercise is essential for the attainment and maintenance of a healthy and symptom-free back, particularly exercises that stress development of muscle strength and flexibility.

What is of more national—indeed international—importance and of personal concern to many is the possible preventive influence of activity on the chances of developing cancer, arthritis, atherosclerotic circuatory diesease (myocardinal infarction, sudden fatal heart rhythm disturbances, strokes or gangrene of the foot, etc.), lung and kidney disease, and a host of other less frequent but individually crippling ailments. A discussion of these conditions follows.

CANCER. There is little conclusive data concerning the cause of cancer, but there is an association of a higher rate of cancer with elevated levels of serum cholesterol—a laboratory finding more usually related to heart disease. The outdoorsman or woman must recognize the potential hazard of sunburn as a cause of skin cancer and apply sunscreens, but otherwise there is little information suggesting a cause and effect relationship between increased activity and malignant disease. In general, exposure to toxic or carcinogenic substances is presumed to be of great importance, and the increased inhalation of some of them with exertion, in either a work or recreational environment, is to be avoided. This, however, does not incriminate the exercise itself. If anything it is reasonable to assume that the more active, and thus, perhaps the more competent set of lungs will have better defenses against noxious exposures. However, we know of no proof that physical training helps prevent bronchitis, emphysema, pneumonia, or lung cancer—except by discouraging the use of tobacco. Moderate exercise is well tolerated by many asthmatics and may help with this disabling condition.

ARTHRITIS. Those who exercise and feel their age through creaking and painful joints would like to be reassured that maintaining a certain activity level will help retard or arrest the progressive arthritic degeneration of advancing years. Many of us believe a good activity program helps, but there are no definitive studies that tell us what activities in youth, middle years, and later will provide optimal defense against arthritic damage. A Veterans Administration record review suggests that deep knee bends in training camp were associated with more knee disorders later in life, and there is even more concern about "Little League Elbow" leading to later complaints. Both of these problems, however, can be avoided by a cutback in the frequency of the specific activity.

HEART DISEASE. It is in the area of heart disease that both the most interest and the most controversy exists—perhaps because diseases of the circulation are responsible for more than 50 percent of deaths in the United States and many developed countries.

Among circulatory diseases there can be a division made between those of the heart itself and the coronary arteries and those of the blood vessels—the peripheral vascular system.

PERIPHERAL VASCULAR DISEASE. It is widely accepted, although more on a basis of individual patient observations than the result of controlled clinical trials, that varicose vein disease of the legs also responds well to exercise, with or without elastic support hose. For some people surgical removal of large varicosities is indicated, but active leg exercise will help many and even decrease the unsightly appearance of some distended veins. Weight lifting and long intervals of standing or sitting should be replaced by activities such as stair climbing, dancing, tennis, bicycle riding, and particularly swimming. The support of the cool water is proportional to the forces of gravity within the vein, and the adrenalin response of exercise and the cold will help stimulate a contraction of the muscle in the vein wall.

Thrombophlebitis (clotting of the veins) and its complications of clots being carried to the lungs (embolism) are less likely to occur in individuals who are habitually active, unless they are injured or immobilized by imprudent actions.

CORONARY HEART DISEASE. Coronary heart disease is presently the Achilles heel of the American population relative to disability and death. Cardiovascular diseases, of which coronary heart disease is the most severe, accounted for 994,513 deaths in the United States in 1975 (see Figure 1.1). This represented over 53 percent of deaths from all causes. In other words, cardiovascular disease alone accounted for more of the total number of deaths in the United States in 1975 than the combined total of all other causes of death! Of this total number of deaths due to cardiovascular disease, 642,719 or 64.6 percent were the result of heart attack. Therefore, heart attack alone accounts

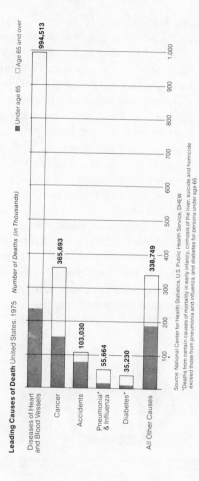

FIGURE 1.1. Causes of death in the United States during the year 1975. (Courtesy of American Heart Association. *Heart Facts—1978.* American Heart Association, Dallas, 1977.)

for nearly 35 percent of all deaths in this country. Heart and blood vessel diseases cost our nation an estimated $28.5 billion each year, in addition to lost income and a loss of an estimated 52 million man-days of production each year.

Among American males between age 33 and 65—the years when both family and society depend on a man's productivity—coronary heart disease causes one-third of the deaths. For approximately every coronary death in the United States there is a more fortunate survivor who will need emotional and physical rehabilitation. Both groups have added up to almost a million and one-half coronary events each year. Recently a slight but definite trend for fewer coronary deaths has become recognized—perhaps because of risk factor modification and the increase in personal physical activity. Even a 10 percent annual reduction in "coronaries" would provide increased taxes and decreased medical care costs far in excess of the entire research budget of the National Heart, Lung and Blood Institute, not to speak of savings in terms of personal and family distress.

Coronary heart disease is the result of atherosclerosis, which is a slow, progressive disease where the inside linings of the arteries become thickened by deposits of fat, fibrin, cellular debris, and calcium. This thickening causes the arteries to lose their pliability, and the channel through which the blood is transported becomes narrowed, restricting normal blood flow in its more advanced stages. In the case of coronary

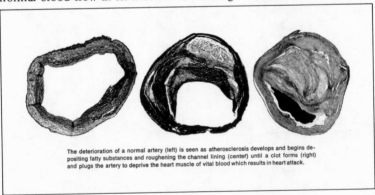

The deterioration of a normal artery (left) is seen as atherosclerosis develops and begins depositing fatty substances and roughening the channel lining (center) until a clot forms (right) and plugs the artery to deprive the heart muscle of vital blood which results in heart attack.

FIGURE 1.2. Progression of coronary atherosclerosis. (Courtesy of American Heart Association. *Heart Facts—1978.* American Heart Association, Dallas, 1977.

heart disease, the coronary vessels that supply the heart become narrowed, and when one of the vessels becomes blocked by a blood clot, the result is a heart attack (see Figure 1.2). The severity of the heart attack is determined by the location of the blockage, since that part of the heart muscle supplied by the blocked artery does not get sufficient oxygen and nutrients and begins to die.

The narrowing of the coronary arteries is a long, slow process that begins very early in life. Kannel and Dawber have recently stated that atherosclerosis is not only a disease of the aged but also is primarily a pediatric problem, since the pathological changes that lead to atherosclerosis begin in infancy and progress during childhood. Enos and others found that 70 percent of autopsied Korean War combat casualties, with an average age of 22.1 years, already had at least moderately advanced coronary atherosclerosis. In a more recent study, McNamara and others found evidence of atherosclerosis in 45 percent of Vietnam War casualties, with 5 percent demonstrating severe coronary atherosclerosis. Fatty streaks or lipid (fat) deposits in the walls of the coronary vessels, which are considered to be the probable precursor to fibrous plaques, are common in children by the age of three to five years. This points to the need to begin preventive programs as early in life as possible.

Over the past 20 to 25 years, researchers have attempted to determine the basic cause of the atherosclerotic process. One approach to gaining a better understanding of the disease is to observe large populations over long periods of time and to determine what those who die from coronary heart disease have in common. As a result of these population studies, certain factors have been identified which, when present, place the individual at an increased risk for the premature or advanced development of coronary heart disease. These factors include the following.

Factors that cannot be altered

- Heredity.
- Sex.
- Race.
- Age.

Factors that can be altered

- Cigarette smoking (and possibly other tobacco use).
- Hypertension (high blood pressure).
- Elevated serum cholesterol, triglyceride, and levels of low-density lipoproteins.
- Diet (as associated with saturated fat intake and obesity).
- Physical inactivity.
- Obesity/Adiposity (body fatness).
- Diabetes.
- Emotional stress.
- Electrocardiogram abnormalities.

The three primary or major risk factors are hypertension, elevated serum cholesterol levels, and cigarette smoking. The risks associated with these three factors, singly and in combination, are illustrated in Figure 1.3. It is important to note that a combination of all three primary risk factors leads to a 3.8 times greater risk of heart attack. In a recent study of coronary heart disease risk factors in 8- to 12-year-old boys, 36 percent exhibited no risk factors, 46 percent had one, and 18 percent had two or more.

HYPERTENSION. Hypertension is a disease that is the result of an unstable or persistent elevation of blood pressure above the normal range. Unfortunately, hypertension is often a silent disease, that is, there are no characteristic symptoms. It is also a puzzling disease, since the cause is unknown in over 90 percent of the cases, and there is no cure, although the disease can be controlled through medication, weight reduction, diet, and exercise. It is estimated that hypertension was present in 24,080,000 people in this country during the year 1975. It can lead to death or disability through stroke, congestive heart failure, and kidney failure, and it is a major risk factor in coronary heart disease.

The role of exercise in hypertension is unclear at the present time. It does appear that those individuals who are physically active have a lower incidence of hypertension when compared to those who are sedentary. Likewise, systolic and diastolic blood pressures have been lowered in individuals who were hypertensive, as a result of a formal physical training program. Few, if any, changes have been noted in individuals whose blood pressures were considered normal prior to participation in an activity program.

These charts show the extent to which particular risk factors increased the risk of heart attack and stroke in the male population, aged 30-62 of Framingham, Mass. For each disease, columns below the black horizontal line indicate lower than average risk; columns above the line, higher than average risk.

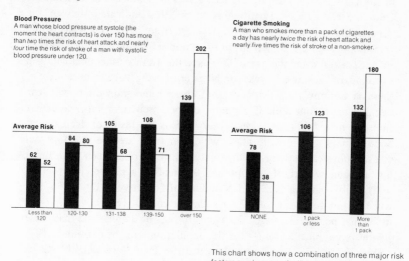

Blood Pressure
A man whose blood pressure at systole (the moment the heart contracts) is over 150 has more than *two* times the risk of heart attack and nearly *four* time the risk of stroke of a man with systolic blood pressure under 120.

Cigarette Smoking
A man who smokes more than a pack of cigarettes a day has nearly *twice* the risk of heart attack and nearly *five* times the risk of stroke of a non-smoker.

This chart shows how a combination of three major risk factors can increase the likelihood of heart attack and stroke. For purposes of illustration, this chart uses an abnormal blood pressure level of 180 systolic, and a cholesterol level of 310 in a 45-year old man.

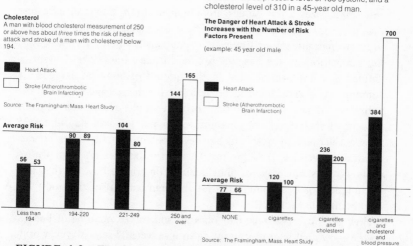

Cholesterol
A man with blood cholesterol measurement of 250 or above has about *three* times the risk of heart attack and stroke of a man with cholesterol below 194.

Source: The Framingham, Mass. Heart Study

The Danger of Heart Attack & Stroke Increases with the Number of Risk Factors Present

(example: 45 year old male

Source: The Framingham, Mass. Heart Study

FIGURE 1.3. Figure shows increased risk of heart attack or stroke with one or more of the primary-risk factors. (Courtesy of American Heart Association. *Heart Facts–1978.* American Heart Association, Dallas, 1977.)

OBESITY. Obesity has become a problem of epidemic proportions in the United States during the past several decades. Statistics from the United States Public Health Service in 1966 indicated that of the American population over 30 years of age, from 25 to 46 percent of the total population are 20 percent or more above their best or ideal weight. In both sexes, after the age of 25 years, the average individual will gain 1 pound of weight per year, or 10 pounds every decade. In addition, there is accumulating evidence that these same individuals will lose one-quarter to one-half of a pound of lean weight or fat-free weight (muscle, bone, skin, etc.) each year. This is the result of decreases in bone mineral and muscle mass, which, in turn, are the result of decreased physical activity. With a net gain of 1 pound each year and a loss in lean weight of one-quarter to one-half a pound, the average individual is gaining 1.25 to 1.5 pounds of fat per year. By age 55, this will amount to a gain of 37.5 to 45.0 pounds of fat, above what the individual possessed at age 25. Again, it must be emphasized that these figures represent the average for the population, not the extremes.

What is "obesity," and how does it differ from "overweight?" Overweight is defined as body weight that exceeds the normal or standard weight allowed for a particular individual, on the basis of sex, height, and frame size. These values are obtained from standardized tables that have been established on the basis of population averages. Thus, to be overweight, means simply that you exceed the average weight of the population on the basis of sex, height, and frame size. Obesity is defined as being overfat, that is, the amount of body fat exceeds the amount that is considered to be desirable for the sex and weight of the individual. Males should maintain their fat weight at less than 16 to 19 percent of their total body weight, and females should stay under 25 percent. Because of bust and hip development related to sex characteristics in females, they are on the average fatter than men. Unfortunately, it is not easy for individuals to determine how fat they are. Techniques for determining the fat and lean content of the body will be presented in Section 3.

How does exercise relate to obesity, and can exercise be of benefit to the individual who is attempting to lose weight? Jean Mayer, world-famous scientist and nutritionist, has stated that he is, ". . . . convinced that inactivity is the most important factor explaining the frequency of 'creeping' overweight in modern societies." Many experimental studies, using humans as well as animals, have demonstrated a strong, direct link between obesity and physical inactivity. For those attempting to lose weight, fat weight specifically, exercise has been found to be most effective, and in fact, may be the single most important aspect of a weight control program for insuring permanent weight loss. This area will be discussed in much greater detail in Section 2.

PHYSICAL INACTIVITY AS A RISK FACTOR. As yet there is no conclusive proof that stopping smoking and treating high blood pressure, high serum cholesterol, or diabetes will retard the formation or reverse the effect of obstructive fatty deposits in the coronary arteries or elsewhere. The Veterans Administration study of Dr. Fries and colleagues demonstrated the value of antihypertensive therapy in decreasing other blood vessel damage, but there were too few coronary events to demonstrate a difference there. Thus, the preventive approach to coronary disease still needs wide-ranging research including a study of the influence of physical activity: does it precipitate heart attacks, help people to avoid them, or help them survive an attack with less damage?

Before examining the data on heart attack incidence and mortality, it is of interest to evaluate the effects of increased physical activity within a larger context encompassing the following disciplines.

PHYSIOLOGY: Are circulatory reserves reinforced and capabilities increased by physical training?

PSYCHOLOGY: Are those who are active likely to feel better, be more optimistic, be more creative, and have more mental stamina and productivity than those who are sedentary?

EPIDEMIOLOGY: Are physically active persons less likely to develop heart disease at a given age (incidence), be disabled by it (morbidity), or have a fatal outcome (mortality)?

Some of the physiologic changes that accompany physical training are:

A slower heart rate at any submaximal work load after training.

A lower systolic and diastolic blood pressure in many persons at a given submaximal work load.

A greater extraction of oxygen from the total circulating blood.

An ability to pump a larger volume of blood with each contraction of the heart chambers (greater stroke volume expansion).

Increased efficiency leading to a lower heart work demand (power or fuel requirement) for any given external task.

Increased aerobic capacity—resulting from the ability to supply the body with more oxygen and other fuels.

For those who enjoy the physically active life, these enhanced capabilities are highly desirable. Among the inactive population, however, there are many who ask the pertinent question: "Fitness for what?" They claim that they have no need or desire to exercise regularly other than to meet the demands of daily living—taking out the trash, bringing in the groceries, and occasionally shoveling snow. For these persons, sex may no longer be undertaken with much vigor, and sport activities do not extend beyond sporadic soft ball, touch football, social doubles tennis, or skiing. Whatever one thinks of such an attitude, it would help us all if we could find other benefits to be derived from exercise beyond the subjective element of "fun."

An increasing number of psychologists and psychiatrists include physical activities as part of their therapy—both to help recovery from mental illness and to prevent relapses. Many individuals believe they maintain a more positive mental attitude if they get regular physical activity. Dr. Fred Heinzelmann and colleagues developed impressive data in two studies including large populations. The first, known as the Three University Pilot Study, was an effort at Pennsylvania State University and the Universities of Minnesota and Wisconsin to determine if a primary preventive heart disease study of physical activity among "high-risk" but so called "healthy" noncardiac males could be mounted. Forty percent of these men randomly assigned to the "active" group reported that they had more adequate sleep and rest during the program, while there was a negligible change reported by those in the control group. The "active" men reported a decreased amount of total food intake and found time for extra recreation outside the program, even though they were told to maintain the same lifestyle as before the exercise program started. Even more striking was the finding that the "active" men had less perceived "stress and tension" and experienced "feelings of better health" and increased "stamina" than their more sedentary colleagues. They also lost more body weight.

Of interest relative to socioeconomic values is the fact that the "active" group reported a sense of increased "work performance" and also a "more positive reaction to work," while the nonactive group reported almost no change.

A study from the Division of Occupational Health at the National Aeronautics and Space Administration reported the enhancement of the same measures of habits, behavior, health, and work, and demonstrated a direct relationship between the frequency of exercise sessions attended and measures of perceived benefit. Thus there is considerable research evidence to support the concept that the quality of life is improved by a well-tolerated program of increased physical acitivity.

Epidemiology, the study of the circumstances in which disease occurs, is a demanding scientific discipline often requiring large numbers of subjects observed over many years. Through "observational epidemiology," cause and effect relationships have been suggested linking given characteristics with an altered disease pattern. Proof often has to depend on "experimental epidemiology" to convince the appropriately skeptical scientific community that such a relationship actually exists. The "controlled trial," with random assignment of individuals to different management programs, may be necessary to prove that a given change in circumstances will affect that person's chances for better health.

What has been found concerning physical activity and the occurrence and severity of heart disease? In their comparison of bus drivers and bus conductors, Professor J.N. Morris of London and colleagues brought forth the first large-scale body of data in 1953. They found that the physically more active conductors had a 30 percent lesser occurrence of all manifestations of coronary heart disease and 50 percent fewer myocardial infarctions. Mortality from coronary heart disease was less than half as frequent in the conductors. A similar finding was found by the same investigators among postal workers delivering mail when compared with less active postal service clerks.

Morris and his associates followed their earlier publication with a 1956 report entitled "Physique of Busmen: The Epidemiology of Uniforms." For any given height, the drivers, upon entry into the transport system, were fitted with trousers having at least a one-inch greater waist circumference than the conductors. The drivers were also found to have higher serum cholesterol and blood pressure levels. Because the groups were already different upon entry into the system, it is difficult to determine if the greater physical activity of the conductors helped lower these levels or if these individuals were indeed different (less fat, etc.) before entry into the service.

Many other observational studies were sparked by Morris's provocative reports. The majority of these studies show a *lesser age–specific rate of coronary disease* in the *more active* groups. The disease was also found to be less severe and accompanied by a lower mortality rate in those groups.

The *amount* and *level* of activity that appears to provide this protection against coronary disease is of great interest. Is it possible, within a time-pressured modern life, to acquire the presumed benefits by engaging in some not too demanding activities that are themselves rewarding and preferably fun? Relative to this important question, the following studies are of interest.

In North Dakota, Dr. Zukel demonstrated a significant relationship between the incidence of coronary heart disease and hours of heavy labor. His data revealed that people who engaged in from one to two hours of heavy physical labor per day had less than one-fifth the incidence of coronary events as those whose usual life pattern included no heavy work. Unfortunately, this data did not permit an analysis for less than one hour per day.

The large (55,000 men) study of the Health Insurance Program of urban New York also produced some encouraging results. The main difference in the incidence of heart attack deaths occurred between the "least active" and the "moderately active" groups. The few extra blocks of walking, extra stair climbing and other activities of the "moderately active" group appeared to help protect them from heart attack deaths, and suggests the potential for useful increased activity without a great change in life-style.

There are those who state that one can achieve complete "immunity" from fatal heart attacks by running at least 6 miles, three times a week, or by frequent involvement in 26-plus mile marathon runs. Even if such were the case, however, it appears unlikely that most citizens will rise to this level of commitment. However, Skinner and colleagues calculated that daily caloric expenditure increases of 400 to 500 calories were associated with a significantly lesser prevalence of coronary heart disease in the multiracial communities of Evans County, Georgia. Taylor reported a similar figure for railroad workers.

Geoffrey Rose of Britain reported that walking 20 minutes or more to work was associated with a one-third lower incidence of "ischemic-type" (evidence of poor heart blood supply) electrocardiographic abnormalities. Paffenbarger and associates found a 25-percent reduction in coronary heart disease death rates with a 925-calorie-per-day increased energy expenditure among longshoremen.

The most comprehensive study on leisure activities has been by the same pioneer, Professor Morris of London. He and his colleagues compared the appearance of heart attacks in 16,882 40- to 64-year-old British male executive-grade civil servants in relation to the amounts of leisure-time physical activity. They concluded:

> *In men recording vigorous exercise the relative risk of developing coronary disease was about a third that in comparable men who did not, and in men reporting much of it still less. Lighter exercise, and provisional estimates of overall activity, showed no such advantage. Vigorous exercise apparently protected against rapidly fatal heart attacks and other first clinical attacks of coronary disease alike, throughout middle age. The smoking habits of men engaged in such activity were similar to those of the other men in the study.*

Among many interesting and relevant studies, two more deserve mention. Brown and associates found the manifestations of coronary disease in men over 65 to be less among those whose life-time activity patterns placed them in a relatively more active group as compared to their more sedentary colleagues. Although this report suggests a later years' advantage, Kahn's review of postal workers in Washington, D.C. suggests that the difference in the incidence of coronary heart disease became indistinguishable within five years after an individual left the physically more active occupational status. Kahn stated: "there is a suggestion here that physical activity of 5, 10 or 15 years ago may not be associated with change in current mortality risks." Thus, it appears that the potential benefits from physical activity cannot be stored. Exercise habits should be continued regularly if benefits are to be retained.

Cooper and others, in a cross-sectional study on 3000 men, found a significant relationship between the level of cardiorespiratory fitness and selected risk factors and fitness variables (serum cholsterol, triglycerides, glucose and uric acid, systolic blood pressure, percent body fat and weight, resting heart rate, and forced vital capacity), suggesting that those with high cardiorespiratory fitness levels are at a lower risk for the premature development of coronary heart disease.

In summary, after reviewing the current medical research literature on this topic, Dr. William B. Kannel concluded in an editorial for the *New England Journal of Medicine:*

> *Over the years, except for diet, little has been more subject to faddism than physical culture. With the proportion of virtually motionless persons in the general population growing, the need to regain the habit of walking and climbing stairs seems urgent. This conservative approach appears indicated until better means for assessing physical fitness in the office and more trained manpower to supervise prescribed exercise becomes available. It is time to consider engineering physical activity back into daily living to counter the sloth and gluttony promulgated by modern technology and changing mores.*

With the increasing emphasis on *fitness*, it may be more healthy to *remain physically active* than just to achieve a certain fitness standard that may require only infrequent activity for those with superior "genetic endowment."

Research has also shown that endurance-training regimens involving running, fast walking, bicycling, and swimming directly affect many of the risk factors associated with coronary heart disease. Reductions in body weight and fat, blood pressure, serum lipids (mainly triglycerides), and blood sugar, and an increase in the efficiency of the cardiorespiratory system to perform work result from such regimens. Fox, Naughton, and Haskell have listed many of the mechanisms by which exercise may reduce the occurrence or severity of coronary heart disease. The effects may be on the atherosclerotic process directly or on what happens after the fatty material is accumulated on the inner surface of the arteries (see Table 1.1). The authors emphasized the point that exercise *may* reduce the occurrence or severity of coronary heart disease. Conflicting reports concerning many of the items listed make conclusions indefinite at this time.

Coronary collaterals, or natural bypass channels, have become more prominent in some exercised animals after constrictions had been produced in the coronaries themselves. This result has not been found often in the few short-term studies that have been performed on humans. Nor have vessels been shown to enlarge to the unusually great size found by Drs. Currens and Paul Dudley White in the famous runner Clarence DeMar who died of cancer at age 69, two years after running his last Boston Marathon.

TABLE 1.1. Mechanisms by which physical activity may reduce the occurrance or severity of coronary heart disease[a]

INCREASE	DECREASE
Coronary collateral vascularization	Serum lipid levels
Vessel size	Triglycerides
Myocardial efficiency	Cholesterol
Efficiency of peripheral blood distribution and return	Glucose intolerance
Electron transport capacity	Obesity-adiposity
Fibrinolytic capability	Platelet stickiness
Red blood cell mass and blood volume	Arterial blood pressure
Thyroid function	Heart rate
Growth hormone production	Vulnerability to dysrhythmias
Tolerance to stress	Neurohormonal overreaction
Prudent living habits	"Strain" associated with
"Joie de vivre"	psychic "stress"

[a]From S.M. Fox, J.P. Naughton, and W.L. Haskell. *Ann. Clin. Res., 3*:404-432 (1971).

Efficiency of the myocardium and blood distribution are not easily studied in humans. If these factors are increased through exercise or physical training, however, they would hold considerable preventive value in improving the individual's ability to survive the stress of an accident, psychological challenge, or heart attack.

Enhancement of one's tolerance to stress would be most desirable in this time-pressured and complex world. Many individuals feel more able to "cope" effectively when they are getting regular exercise. Measurement of "stress" and "strain" have been difficult, however, and studies to date have not been considered adequate.

"Joie de vivre" is a delightful French expression that means more than merely the "joy of living." Enthusiasm, optimism, and bouyancy are all implied within the term. Perhaps these are the elements that allegedly prompted Mae West to say it was not so much "the men in her life" that mattered as "the life in her man."

Serum triglyceride levels decrease after physical exertion in most people and continue to lower for one and one-half to two days. Some studies have implicated the triglyceride fraction of serum lipids in the background of coronary disease, although the risk relationship is not as strong as with serum cholesterol elevation. Some investigators have found lower cholesterol levels to result from exercise, often in association with reduction in body weight. However, the cholesterol decline in most of these reports, has been modest, and there are others demonstrating no significant change. Lopez and associates have indicated that an exercise program will reduce the apparently hazardous *low-density* lipoprotein fraction with an almost equivalent rise in the *high-density* fraction, thought by many to be neutral or possibly protective. This fascinating refinement in our insight into fat metabolism may be of considerable long-term significance in our preventive efforts.

Although many individuals remember having a large appetite after physical activity, there is evidence that appetite is actually supressed for 30 to 90 minutes after exertion.

The need to support an elevated blood pressure or a faster than optimal heart rate requires more heart power and therefore greater fuel supplies for a specific task. Hence, in reducing heart rate and blood pressure, physical training insures that greater reserves are available in case of accident or heart damage. A greater peak capacity will also be available without excessive heart rate, blood pressure, or power demands. Although there are no conclusive studies proving the value of increased physical activity in the treatment of hypertension, it is well-established that the elevated blood pressure obtained during exercise tolerance testing before a physical-conditioning program will be reduced upon evaluation after an effective program.

Blackburn and associates found a reduced number of premature electrocardiographic complexes in exercising men as compared to more sedentary controls. This suggests a possible decrease in the susceptibility of the heart to catastrophic rhythm disturbances. Perhaps this is due to decreased "neurohormonal over-reaction" or a lesser production of adrenaline related substances known as catecholamines.

Although there is conflicting evidence concerning the mechanisms by which physical activity may prevent diseases of the heart, the role of exercise appears promising. The need exists to explore the long-range effects of exercise on the risk factors and incidence of coronary heart disease.

Much has been written on these aspects, and a significant amount remains to be learned. Nevertheless, there are many reasons to accept what the epidemiologic studies suggest: those who are physically more active have less disease at a given age, what they have is less severe, and less frequently fatal. We have not yet supplied proof of the cost effectiveness of physical activity programs, either to the individual or to the community. The physiological improvement, however, is so well-established that it is considered predictable in almost anyone who becomes more active.

In any case, the chief reason why most of us continue our exercise programs is, quite simply, because we feel better, perform better, and find greater enjoyment in a higher quality of life.

A MORE ACTIVE LIFE-STYLE: A BASIC NEED OF MODERN MEN AND WOMEN

Our modern life-style has channeled each of us into an increasingly sedentary existence. "Homo sapiens" has been dramatically transformed into "homo sedentarius." Men and women were designed and constructed for movement and vigorous activity and have not adapted well to this sedentary existence. From the above discussion, it is obvious that physical inactivity has very serious implications for the health and well-being of the average individual. Regular exercise must be programmed back into our life-styles. Where the average American used to lead a very active and vigorous life—farming, working in heavy construction, and working in other jobs requiring hard physical labor—the modern American is typically tied to a chair throughout the average workday and goes home "exhausted," only to sit for several more hours in front of the television screen. To counter the changes made by modern technology, exercise must be programmed into our present-day life-style.

Regular exercise is necessary to develop and maintain an optimal level of health, performance, and appearance. Research has shown that regular physical exercise enhances the function of the joints; increases the sense of physical well-being and promotes a sense of "feeling good;" increases physical working capacity by increasing cardiorespiratory fitness and muscle strength and endurance; and decreases the risk of serious diseases that could lead to early disability and death. In addition, physical activity provides an outlet for the dissipation of tension and mental fatigue, aids in weight reduction and control, improves posture, contributes to a youthful appearance, enhances one's self-image, and increases general vitality. In short, regular exercise of a vigorous nature has much to offer those who have been leading a sedentary life and who have watched themselves deteriorate over the years. However, it must be carried on as a life-time pursuit, since the benefits rapidly disappear once training is stopped.

DESIGNED EXERCISE PROGRAMS FOR THE INDIVIDUAL

In the past, exercise programs were designed on a group basis. Each person in the group would attempt to perform exactly the same exercises and at the same rate as everyone else in the group. It finally became obvious that when everyone is put through the same program at the same pace, each person is working at a different percentage of his or her capacity, that is, some are working at full capacity and cannot maintain the pace, while others are working at a rate that is well below their capacity. As a result, a concerted effort was initiated to develop a sound and rational basis for designing exercise programs for the individual. Through a review of past research and a launching of new, well-designed research programs, the art of prescribing exercise began to develop a scientific basis. It was at this point that exercise was prescribed on an individual basis, taking into consideration individual differences in abilities, capacities, and likes and dislikes.

The foundation of an individualized exercise program is the comprehensive medical examination and fitness profile that is strongly recommended for any adult before starting an exercise program. The medical examination should include a thorough family and personal medical history, a physical examination, resting blood pressure and electrocardiogram, blood analyses for fasting blood sugar and blood fats (cholesterol and triglyceride), and an exercise electrocardiogram, taken while the individual exercises to volitional fatigue. Details of the medical examination will be presented in Section 3. The fitness profile begins where the medical examination ends. The medical examination reveals the absence or presence of a disease or poor health, while the fitness profile indicates the degree of health. Dr. Robert K. Kerlan, well-known sports physician and orthopedic consultant, refers to the medical examination as rating the individual on a "0" to "−100" scale, "0" representing absence of disease and "−100" representing death. He proposes that the fitness profile rate the individual on a "0" to "+100" basis, "0" representing the absence of disease with a lack of vitality, vigor, and other positive health attributes, and "+100" representing perfect health. The fitness profile typically evaluates the individual's working capacity or cardiorespiratory fitness level, body composition (fat and lean weight), flexibility, and strength and muscular endurance. Once the individual has received medical clearance and has had a fitness profile established, it is then possible to accurately design an exercise program, tailored to the needs, interests, and abilities of that individual. Thus, a fitness profile is important to properly classify one's capacity and level of ability, as well as to have a baseline for future comparison. Details of the physical fitness profile will also be presented in Section 3.

When prescribing exercise for the individual, five factors are to be considered: type or mode of activity, frequency of participation, duration of participation, intensity of participation, and initial level of fitness. The primary activity should be of an endurance nature such as walking, jogging, running, swimming, bicycling, or hiking. Secondary activities should emphasize the development of strength, muscular endurance, and flexibility. It is important to select activities that the individual will enjoy and be willing to pursue. The endurance conditioning benefits gained from tennis are not nearly as great as those gained from jogging or running, but if the participant dislikes jogging and enjoys tennis, tennis is the activity that should be prescribed, even though it may take him or her longer to gain the same endurance benefits. Exercise must be viewed as a life-time pursuit, and therefore attractive activities must be made available.

For individuals with a low initial endurance capacity, it is advisable to prescribe an activity such as walking or jogging for the first three to six months. Once the desired endurance level is reached, the individual can be placed on a maintenance program using game or recreational activities such as tennis, handball, racketball, and badminton. It is far better to get into shape before playing a specific sport, rather than trying to use the sport as the vehicle for getting into shape.

Relative to exercise duration and frequency, it appears that 3 to 5 days per week at 20 to 60 minutes per day of endurance exercise is optimal. This is not to say that longer or more frequent exercise sessions wouldn't result in greater improvement, for they will. It simply implies that to invest additional time above that suggested as optimal will produce smaller gains for the extra time invested. With respect to the intensity of exercise, it appears that there may be a minimal level or threshold, below which a conditioning effect will not occur. This is approximately 50 percent of the participants' endurance capacity, although there is a great deal of individual variation. A training intensity of 50 to 80 percent of one's endurance capacity (maximum oxygen uptake) appears to be optimal. This can be easily monitored and controlled by the participant, by determining the heart rate equivalent to the selected working intensity. The participant then monitors his or her pulse rate during exercise to keep it at this training level. This is referred to as the training heart rate. The training heart rate can be determined from the information ascertained from the exercise stress test. Section 4 will consider the concept of exercise prescription in more detail.

GENERAL CONCEPTS IN EXERCISE PRESCRIPTION

Exercise serves many purposes and has specific outcomes that are totally dependent on the type of exercise performed. The shot putter who trains with weights is exercising to gain strength to improve the distance he or she can put the shot. The sprinter who trains by running 100-yard sprints at near maximal speed is exercising to increase speed. The middle-aged person who performs a series of calisthenic-type back exercises is attempting to gain flexibility and strength to overcome constant pain and discomfort in the lower back area. Middle-aged joggers desire to improve or maintain their present level of health and are improving the functioning of their cardiovascular and respiratory systems. Thus training is highly specific, that is, the purpose, goals, and outcome are largely dependent on the nature of the activity.

Exercise works on specific aspects or components of the body or of the body functions. These can be categorized into two general areas, as follows.

Health-Related Components

○ Cardiorespiratory endurance

○ Muscular strength and endurance

○ Flexibility

○ Body composition

○ Relaxation and emotional stability

○ Risk factor reduction

Performance-Related Components

○ Cardiorespiratory endurance

○ Muscular strength, power, and endurance

○ Flexibility

○ Body composition

○ Agility

○ Speed

○ Neuromuscular coordination

○ Specific skill

This book is concerned mainly with the health-related components even though there is considerable overlap between the two areas.

When exercise is undertaken primarily for the health-related benefits, the primary emphasis must be placed on the development of cardiorespiratory endurance. General muscular strength, muscular endurance, and flexibility are also important and need to be integrated into the individual's total exercise program. As mentioned earlier, activities such as brisk walking, jogging, running, bicycling, and swimming are appropriate for the development of cardiorespiratory endurance. Traditional calisthenic-type exercise programs are appropriate for developing flexibility, strength, and muscular endurance, but have little, if any, effect on the development of cardiorespiratory endurance Therefore, when designing an exercise program, it is important to define the major purpose of the program, for example, general health, and then to select the activities accordingly. The outcome of the exercise program is dependent on the type of exercise or exercises selected. This is referred to as the specificity of training.

Two additional and related concepts of importance in designing exercise programs are the concepts of "overload" and "progressive resistance exercise." Although these two terms were originally restricted in use to the area of weight training, they are appropriate for conditioning in all areas. Overload refers to the need of the individual to stress the body, or one or more of its parts or systems, above those levels normally encountered. As an example, a worker on an assembly line must remove a 75-pound object from a conveyor belt and place it into a packing carton. For his first few days on the job, this represents a considerable stress and taxes his muscles to near capacity. As a result, his muscles increase in strength up to a point where this task is handled with ease, a process that could take several months. At this point, however, the muscle strength levels off and does not continue to increase. If the factory suddenly shifted to 90-pound objects, this would constitute a new overload, and he would then continue to gain in strength. Thus, the muscles must be taxed beyond so-called "normal" levels of work in order for significant increases in strength to occur. The same principle holds for the development of flexibility, cardiorespiratory endurance, or any other health-related or performance-related component.

Progressive resistance exercise is also illustrated in the above example. As the muscles become stronger, or as the individual becomes better conditioned, it takes a proportionately greater stress to continue improvement. In essence, this is the systematic application of the overload principle.

SUMMARY

Human beings have grown increasingly sedentary with the advancement of technology. Adoption of this new life-style has resulted in a new category of disease, termed hypokinetic disease (diseases resulting from the lack of exercise), which is directly or indirectly the result of physical inactivity, and includes coronary heart disease, hypertension, obesity, anxiety and depression, and lower back problems. Each of these was discussed and their link to physical inactivity was established.

In order to combat the trend toward physical inactivity, increasing attention has been given to study and research in the exercise sciences to evaluate various approaches to exercise and to determine how to best motivate the general population to participate in regular exercise. From this, the concept of an individualized exercise program has evolved. The individualized exercise program is prescribed on the basis of a comprehensive medical examination and fitness profile. Factors considered in the prescription include type or mode of activity, frequency, duration, intensity of participation, and initial level of fitness. General factors in prescribing exercise were then discussed, including specificity of training, the overload principle, and the principle of progressive resistance exercise.

REFERENCES

1. American Heart Association. *Heart Facts—1978.* American Heart Association, Dallas, Tex., 1977.

2. Blackburn, H., H.L. Taylor, B. Hamrell, E. Buskirk, W.C. Nicholas, and R.D. Thorsen. "Premature ventricular complexes induced by stress testing: their frequency and response to physical conditioning." *Am. J. Cardiol., 31*:441-449 (1973).

3. Boyer, J.L., and F.W. Kasch. "Exercise therapy in hypertensive men." *JAMA, 211*:1668-1671 (1970).

4. Brown, R.G., A.G. Davidson, T. McKeown, and A.G.W. Whitfield. "Coronary artery disease: influences affecting its incidence in males in the seventh decade." *Lancet, 2*:1073-1077 (1957).

5. Cooper, K.H., M.L. Pollock, R.P. Martin, S.R. White, A.C. Lin-

nerud, and A. Jackson. "Physical fitness levels versus selected coronary risk factors: A cross-sectional study." *JAMA, 236*: 166-169 (1976).

6. Durbeck, D.C., F. Heinzelmann, J. Schacter, W.L. Haskell, G. Payne, R. Moxley, M. Nemiroff, D. Limoncelli, L. Arnoldi, and S.M. Fox. "The NASA-USPHS health evaluation and enhancement program." *Am. J. Cardiol., 30*:784-790 (1972).

7. Enos, W.F., R.H. Holmes, and J. Beyer. "Coronary disease among United States soldiers killed in action in Korea." *JAMA, 152*: 1090-1093 (1953).

8. Fox, S.M., III, and W.L. Haskell. "Physical activity and the prevention of coronary heart disease." *Bull. NY Acad. Med., 44*:950-967 (1968).

9. Fox, S.M., III, J.P. Naughton, and P.A. Gorman. "Physical activity and cardiovascular disease." *Mod. Conc. Cardiov. Dis., 41*:17-30 (1972).

10. Fox, S.M., III, J.P. Naughton, and W.L. Haskell. "Physical activity and the prevention of coronary heart disease." *Ann. Clin. Res., 3*:404-432 (1971).

11. Friedman, M., and R.M. Rosenmann. *Type A Behavior and Your Heart.* New York; Alfred A. Knopf, 1974.

12. Froelicher, V.F., and A. Oberman. "An analysis of epidemiologic studies of physical inactivity as a risk factor for coronary artery disease." *Progr. Cardiovasc. Dis., 15*:41-65 (1972).

13. Hein, F.V., D.L. Farnsworth, and C.E. Richardson. *Living: Health, Behavior and Environment,* Fifth Edition. Glenview, Ill.: Scott, Foresman, 1970.

14. Heinzelmann, F., and R.W. Bagley. "Response to physical activity programs and their effects on health behavior." *Public Health Rep., 85*:905-911 (1970).

15. Jenkins, C.D. "The coronary-prone personality." In: *Psychological Aspects of Myocardial Infarction and Coronary Care,* W.D. Gentry and R.R. Williams (eds). St. Louis: C.V. Mosby, 1975, p. 5.

16. Kahn, H.A. "The relationship of reported coronary heart disease mortality to physical activity of work." *Am. J. Public Health,*

        53:1058-1067 (1963).

17. Kannel, W.B. "Physical exercise and lethal atherosclerotic disease."
    N. Engl. J. Med., 282:1153-1154 (1970).

18. Kannel, W.B., and T.R. Dawber. "Atherosclerosis as a pediatric
    problem." *J. Pediatrics, 80*:544-554 (1972).

19. Klatshy, A., G.D. Friedman, A.B. Siegelaub, and M.J. Gerard.
    "Alcohol consumption and blood pressure: Kaiser-Permanente
    multiphasic health examination data." *N. Engl. J. Med., 296*:
    1194-1200 (1977).

20. Kraus, H. *The Cause, Prevention and Treatment of Backache Stress
    and Tension.* New York: Simon & Schuster, 1972.

21. Kraus, H., and A. Melleby. *The Y's Way to a Healthy Back.* YMCA
    of Greater New York, 1976.

22. Kraus, H., and W. Raab. *Hypokinetic Disease.* Springfield, Ill.:
    Charles C. Thomas, 1961.

23. Lutwak, L., and A. Coulston. "Activity and obesity." In: *Obesity
    in Perspective,* G.A. Bray, (ed.). Department of Health, Educa-
    tion and Welfare Publication No. (NIH) 75-708, Washington,
    D.C., 1975.

24. Mayer, J. *Overweight.* Englewood Cliffs, N.J.: Prentice-Hall, 1968.

25. McNamara, J.J., M.A. Molot, J.F. Stremple, and R.T. Cutting.
    "Coronary artery disease in combat casualties in Vietnam."
    JAMA, 216:1185-1187 (1971).

26. Morgan, W.P. *Introduction to Sport Psychology.* St. Louis: C.V.
    Mosby, 1978.

27. Morgan, W.P. "Selected physiological and psychomotor correlates
    of depression in psychiatric patients." *Res. Q., 39*:1037-1043
    (1968).

28. Morris, J.N., J.A. Heady, and P.A.B. Raffle. "Physique of London
    busmen: epidemiology of uniforms." *Lancet, 2*:569-570 (1956).

29. Morris, J.N., J.A. Heady, P.A.B. Raffle, C.G. Roberts, and J.W.
    Parks. "Coronary heart disease and physical activity of work."
    Lancet, 2:1053-1057, 1111-1120 (1953).

30. Morris, J.N., S.P.N. Chave, C. Adams, C. Sirey, and L. Epstein.
    "Vigorous exercise in leisure-time and the incidence of coronary

heart disease." *Lancet, 1*:333-339 (1973).

31. U.S. Public Health Service. *Obesity and Health:* U.S. Government Printing Office, Washington, D.C., 1966.

32. Oscai, L.B. "The role of exercise in weight control." In: *Exercise and Sport Sciences Reviews,* Jack H. Wilmore (ed.), Vol. I. New York: Academic Press, 1973.

33. Paffenbarger, R.S., Jr., M.E. Laughlin, A.S. Gima, and R.A. Black. "Work activity of longshoremen as related to death from coronary heart disease and stroke." *N, Engl. Med., 282*: 1109-1114 (1970).

34. Paffenbarger, R.S., and W.E. Hale. "Work activity and coronary heart mortality." *N. Engl. J. Med., 292*:545-550 (1975).

35. Pitts, F.H., Jr. "Biochemical factors in anxiety neurosis." *Behavioral Sciences, 16*:82-91 (1971).

36. Reville, F.P. "Sport for all: physical activity and the prevention of disease." Council for Cultural Co-operation, Council of Europe, Strasbourg, 1970.

37. Rose, G. "Physical activity and coronary heart disease." *Proc. R. Soc. Med., 62*:1183-1187 (1969).

38. Sanne, H.M., and L. Wilhelmsen. "Physical activity as prevention and therapy in coronary heart disease." *Scan. J. Rehab. Med., 3*:47-56 (1971).

39. Skinner, J.S., H. Benson, J.R. McDonough, and C.G. Hames. "Social status, physical activity, and coronary proneness." *J. Chron. Dis., 19*:773-783 (1966).

40. Taylor, H.L., E. Klepetar, A. Keys, W. Parlin, H. Blackburn, and T. Puchner. "Death rates among physically active and sedentary employees of the railroad industry." *Am. J. Public Health, 52*: 1697-1707 (1962).

41. Wilmore, J.H. "Physical exercise and body composition." In: *The Regulation of the Adipose Tissue Mass* J. Vague and J. Boyer (eds.). New York: American Elsevier Publishing, 1974.

42. Wilmore, J.H., and J.J. McNamara. "prevalence of coronary heart disease risk factors in boys, 8 to 12 years of age." *J. Pediatrics, 84*:527-533 (1974).

43. Wilson, N.L., S.M. Farber, L.D. Kimbrough, and R.H.L. Wilson. "The development and perpetuation of obesity: An overview." In: *Obesity*, N.L. Wilson (ed.). Philadelphia: F.A. Davis, 1969.

44. Wright, H.F., and J.H. Wilmore. "Estimation of relative body fat and lean body weight in a United States Marine Corps population." *Aerosp. Med., 45*:301-306 (1974).

45. Zukel, W.J., R.H. Lewis, P.E. Enterline, R.C. Painter, L.S. Ralston, R.M. Fawcett, A.P. Meredith, and B. Peterson. "A short-term community study of the epidemiology of coronary heart disease." *Am. J. Public Health, 49*: 1630-1639 (1959).

Section 2

Research Findings on Exercise, Health Maintenance and Performance

Here we deal with the research findings associated with different types of exercise training programs and their effects on various physiological functions. Even though the various components of physiological function will be discussed as separate entities, remember that the body functions as a whole, and oftentimes something that affects one bodily system has an effect on the whole. For example, a person who is participating in a jogging program generally would be trying to develop or maintain cardiorespiratory fitness. Jogging would also have an effect on the musculoskeletal system of the legs and trunk, that is, some muscular strength and endurance would be developed in these areas with a possible reduction in flexibility. This particular jogging program may stimulate bone development, and on the other hand, if too strenuous, may cause injury. The mind would also be at work during the jog and could perceive the effort in a positive or negative manner. Hence, one can see the complexity involved in trying to quantify the effects of physical activity on the various bodily systems.

CARDIORESPIRATORY FUNCTION

As mentioned in Section 1, good cardiorespiratory function is dependent upon efficient respiratory (lungs) and cardiovascular (heart and blood vessels) systems. Other important factors would include the quality and quantity of the blood (red blood cell count, blood volume, etc.) and specific cellular components that help the body utilize oxygen during exercise. Since it would be difficult to discuss all physiological components and mechanisms that relate to cardiorespiratory function in this volume, only heart rate and oxygen transport and utilization will be mentioned. For a more complete review see Åstrand and Rodahl, and deVries.

The oxygen transport system is made up of the lungs, which bring in fresh air from the external environment and permit oxygen to move across a membrane system (by diffusion) into the circulation. When oxygen reaches the blood it is picked up within the red blood cells and transported through the arterial portion of the circulatory system to the working cells (diffusion and utilization). End products of cellular metabolism (carbon dioxide and lactic acid) are then transported back through the veins of the circulatory system to the heart and lungs. The heart is the key to the oxygen transport system, since it must continually pump large quantities of blood to all bodily systems.

Pulmonary factors, such as total lung volume and maximum breathing capacity, do not limit endurance performance unless one is severely diseased or is training at altitude. That is, under most conditions and at sea level, arterial blood leaving the heart is approximately 97-percent saturated with oxygen, and therefore most of the limitation to endurance performance depends on the capacity of the heart and circulation, and cellular function.

As shown in Table 2.1, important components of the oxygen transport system improve with endurance training. Cardiac output is the amount of blood pumped out of the heart per minute and is determined by multiplying heart rate by stroke volume (amount of blood pumped out of the heart per beat). The arteriovenous oxygen difference represents the amount of oxygen being utilized by the cells from the arterial blood. Maximum oxygen uptake (aerobic capacity) is the largest amount of oxygen that one can utilize under the most strenuous exercise. Because maximum oxygen uptake generally summarizes what is

TABLE 2.1. The effects of physical activity on cardiorespiratory functions

VARIABLES	UNIT	CHANGE WITH ENDURANCE TRAINING
Maximum oxygen uptake	ml/kg·min[b]	Increase
Maximum cardiac output	L/min[c]	Increase
Maximum heart rate	beats/min	Decrease—unchanged
Maximum stroke volume	ml	Increase
Maximum arteriovenous oxygen difference	ml/100 ml blood	Increase—unchanged
Maximum performance	sec	Decrease[a]
Submaximal heart rate	beats/min	Decrease
Resting heart rate	beats/min	Decrease
Resting blood pressure	mm/Hg[d]	Unchanged—decrease

[a]The performance will improve, that is, performance at a given distance will decrease, and performance on a treadmill or work bicycle will increase.

[b]Milliliters per kilogram of body weight per minute.

[c]Liters per minute.

[d]Millimeters of mercury.

going on in the oxygen transport system (including cellular utilization) during maximum or exhaustive exercise and can be measured rather easily, it has been used as the measure most representative of cardiorespiratory fitness. Because a larger person generally has more muscle mass, and thus the capability of burning more oxygen, aerobic capacity is expressed in milliliters of oxygen per kilogram of body weight per minute (ml/kg · min).

Figure 2.1 shows a champion distance runner taking a treadmill test for determination of maximum oxygen uptake. More details on treadmill test procedures and protocols will be discussed in Section 3. Figure 2.2 shows a comparison of maximum oxygen uptake values of young and middle-aged men of various fitness levels. The illustration clearly shows the difference in aerobic capacity as related to status of fitness and age. Values for women are approximately 10 to 20 percent lower.

Are the basic physical characteristics found in champion runners inherited or developed through years of training? The answer, "A champion must be very selective in the manner in which he chooses his parents," is often used. Actually, both inheritance and training are important. Identical twins have been shown to have similar physical characteristics with about a 20 percent difference in aerobic capacity that can be accounted for by endurance training.

Is there a level of aerobic capacity necessary to attain and maintain an optimal level of cardiorespiratory fitness? It is difficult to set a standard for optimal fitness because a specific level of aerobic capacity for optimal health has not been determined. As shown in Figure 2.2, sedentary middle-aged males characteristically fall below 40 milliliters per kilogram of body weight per minute of oxygen uptake. This value drops to 30 by age 50 to 60. The values of 38 to 45 milliliters per kilogram of body weight per minute would seem a reasonable estimate for ages 20 to 60.

Figure 2.3 shows differences in resting heart rate between sedentary and trained groups of men. This information shows that the endurance runner has a slower, stronger, and thus more efficient heart. The slower heart rate is accompanied by a greater stroke volume. A similar adaptation to training occurs during submaximal work, that is, the heart beats more efficiently at a given work load (slower with an increased stroke volume).

A critical exception to the fact that a lower resting heart rate is

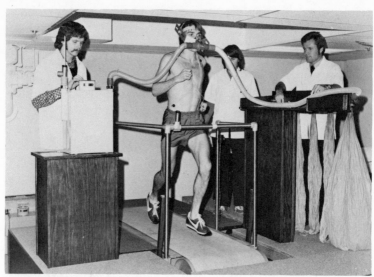

FIGURE 2.1. The maximum oxygen uptake test is being administered to a premier distance runner, the late Steve Prefontaine. At the time of this test, Prefontaine held 10 American distance running records. His maximum oxygen uptake was 84.4 milliliters per kilogram of body weight per minute, one of the highest values ever recorded for a runner. Breathing valve channels all expired air into a series of bags, which were later analyzed for oxygen and carbon dioxide content. Prefontaine was also attached to an electrocardiogram machine by a special 20-foot cable lead system. In this way, the electrical action of the heart and heart rate can be continually monitored throughout the run. It should be noted that more automated systems for determining maximum oxygen uptake are now available.

characteristic of the trained and healthy heart occurs in the case of certain pathologically diseased hearts. In such cases, the heart may beat more slowly permitting a decrease in the metabolic needs of the heart muscle. Another problem in using resting heart rate as a criterion for fitness is its wide variability within the population. For example, Jim Ryan, famous miler, had a high resting heart rate compared to other distance runners (unpublished data: Jack Daniels, University of Texas, Austin). Therefore, caution should be taken when using resting heart rate as a measure of physical fitness. Although women adapt to

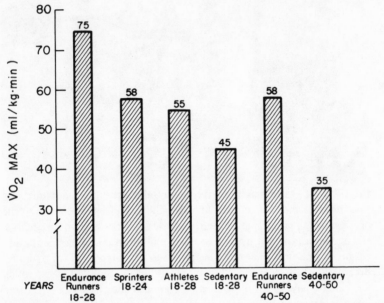

FIGURE 2.2. Comparison of maximum oxygen uptake of young and middle-aged men of various fitness levels.

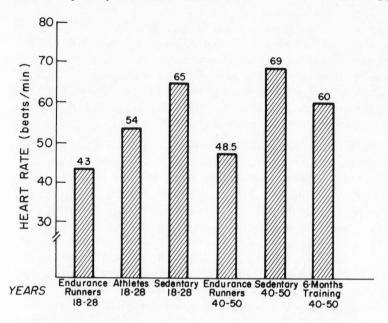

FIGURE 2.3. Comparison of resting heart rate of young and middle-aged men of various fitness levels.

training in the same manner as men, their resting heart rates average 7 to 10 beats per minute higher than men.

Does endurance training reduce blood pressure? If one's blood pressure is generally normal to begin with, physical training has little or no effect on blood pressure reduction. Results from one study using hypertensive patients indicated that exercise significantly lowers blood pressure. Whether or not exercise in itself can normalize blood pressure is still in question. Often a combination of exercise, diet, and medication is necessary for blood pressure control. Caution is necessary for persons who are on blood pressure medication and plan to begin an exercise regimen. Once one begins a program the medication may have to be reduced in order to offset the effect of the training program.

QUANTIFYING THE RESULTS OF ENDURANCE TRAINING PROGRAMS. Improvement in cardiorespiratory fitness is a result of many factors. Generally, the magnitude of improvement is dependent on the total work or energy cost of the exercise regimen. Energy cost can be measured by the number of kilocalories expended, and improvement in cardiorespiratory fitness is dependent upon the intensity, duration, and frequency of the exercise program. Improvement is also related to initial status of health and fitness, mode of exercise, such as walking, running, and cycling, regularity of exercise, and age. These factors, as well as individual interests, should be considered in designing an exercise program to meet the needs and abilities of the person or group involved in the training regimen.

INTENSITY   Two classical studies serve as a practical guide for the determination of a minimal threshold level of intensity for improving aerobic capacity. Both studies agreed that the minimal threshold level for eliciting a training reponse was at a heart rate level equal to approximately 60 percent of the difference between maximal and resting heart rate, that is, maximum heart rate range (approximately 50 percent of maximum aerobic capacity). This method of determining training heart rate is discussed in detail in Section 4. The above heart rate levels ranged from 130 to 150 beats per minute. For unfit individuals and middle-aged and older persons, the minimal training threshold may be as low as 100 to 120 beats per minute. A more recent study by Gledhill and Eynon further substantiates the minimal threshold concept for eliciting a training effect and supports the notion that lower threshold levels are apparent for less fit persons. They trained college men for 10 minutes, five days per week, for five weeks at heart rates of either 120, 135, or 150 beats per minute. When groups were subdivided into low- and high-fitness levels, the high-fitness group showed no improvement at heart rates of 120 beats per minute while the low-fitness group did.

Although the minimal intensity threshold concept described above is generally well accepted, it is also well established that improvement in aerobic capacity is directly related to intensity of training. If training session duration is brief, then low intensity programs may show approximately a 5 percent improvement in aerobic capacity (hardly appreciable), while a high intensity program will elicite a 15 to 20 percent increase.

DURATION   Improvement in cardiorespiratory fitness is also directly related to duration of training. Improvement in aerobic capacity has been shown with moderate to high intensity training lasting only 5 to 10 minutes daily. As a rule, the shorter duration programs (10 to 15 minutes) of moderate intensity show a significantly lower training effect than programs of 30 to 60 minutes duration. Figure 2.4 shows the results from a study conducted on men 20 to 35 years of age for a period of 20 weeks. The intensity was standardized at 85 to 90 percent of maximum heart rate range and the men participated three days per week. Improvement in maximum oxygen uptake was 8.5, 16.1, and 16.8 percent for the 15- , 30- , and 45-minute duration groups, respectively.

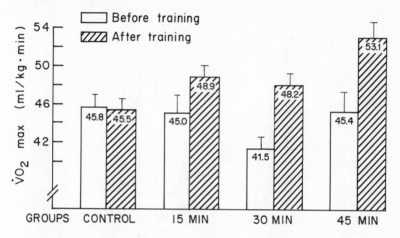

FIGURE 2.4. Effect of different training durations on maximum oxygen uptake ($\dot{V}O_2$ max).

At this stage in the discussion, it is important to emphasize that duration and intensity are closely interrelated, and the notion that the total amount of work (energy cost) accomplished in a training program is an important criterion for fitness development has important implications here. For example, the energy cost of running is generally higher than walking, and yet many men and women would rather walk than run. When the intensity of walking is less than running, can one get similar training effects by the former if duration and frequency are increased? We tried to answer that question several years ago and conducted a 20-week fast-walking study with men 40 to 57 years of age. The men walked for 40 minutes, 4 days per week. The improvement found in this program (Figure 2.5) was equal to that found in 30-minute, 3-day-per-week jogging programs with similarly aged men. The lower intensity of the walking program (65 to 75% of maximum heart rate range) was offset by the increased duration and frequency of training. Thus, the total energy expenditure per week of the two programs was similar.

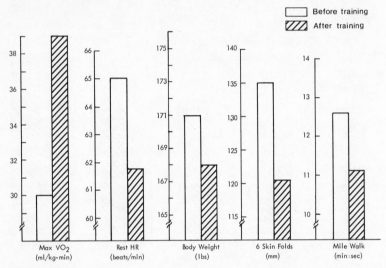

FIGURE 2.5. Effects of walking on the physical fitness of middle-aged men.

When two jogging programs of different intensities (80 versus 90 percent of maximum heart rate range) were compared, the results were similar when total energy expenditure was equalized. This means that participants can slow down their pace, run several minutes longer to make up for the lower calorie expenditure, and end up with approximately the same results.

FREQUENCY Several studies have placed less importance on frequency of training in terms of being as important a training stimulus as intensity or duration. A couple of these investigations have attempted to evaluate frequency by controlling the total number of training sessions or total work output. These studies generally show no difference in aerobic capacity with frequency of training. For example, a group of men were trained for either three or five days per week and, at the end of eight weeks, both groups were re-evaluated. At that time in the experiment, the five-day-per-week group showed more improvement than the three-day group. In an attempt to equalize training sessions (total calorie cost), the three-day-per-week group continued to train another five weeks. Upon re-evaluation, the three-day-per-week group then equalled the improvement of the five-day program. The results of investigations such as this are not surprising, since total energy expenditures were equalized between groups. However, in prescribing exercise, one should not look at frequency of training in this manner because, in reality, training regimens should not terminate after just a few weeks but continue throughout life.

When weeks of training were held constant instead of total number of training sessions, results generally show frequency of training to be a significant factor as a training stimulus. Figure 2.6 shows the results of a training study conducted with men 20 to 35 years of age for a period of 20 weeks. The intensity of training was standardized at 85 to 90 percent of maximum heart rate range with the men participating 30 minutes each exercise session. Improvement in maximum oxygen uptake was 8, 13, and 17 percent for 1- ,3- , and 5-day-per-week training groups.

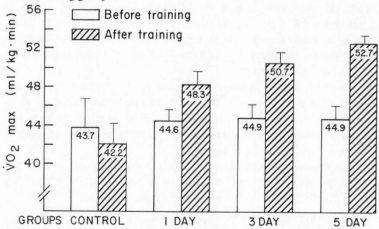

FIGURE 2.6. Effects of different training frequencies on maximum oxygen uptake ($\dot{V}O_2$ max).

Closely related to frequency of training is the regularity at which one continues to participate and its subsequent effect on cardiorespiratory fitness. If training is not continued, the improvements gained in a program diminish rather rapidly. Cureton and Phillips, using equal eight-week periods of training, nontraining, and retraining, found significant improvement, decrement, and improvement, respectively, in cardiorespiratory fitness.

Investigations, whereby subjects are put to bed for extended periods of time, have shown decrements in aerobic capacity and related cardiovascular parameters. Saltin and others confined five subjects to bed for 20 days, followed by a 60-day training period. Cardiovascular efficiency measures regressed during bed rest and improved steadily during training. Table 2.2 shows the results of selected cardiovascular variables.

In an attempt to determine the effects of different magnitudes of detraining, Kendrick re-evaluated 22 middle-aged men after a 12-week detraining period. Participants were originally trained by running 8 miles per week for 20 weeks and were subsequently divided into the following three subgroups: group A continued to train 8+ miles per week, group B trained 3 miles per week, and group C was inactive. The results showed group A to maintain or improve their level of fitness, while groups B and C regressed significantly. Group C lost approximately 50 percent of its original improvement after 12 weeks. Another study showed a complete regression back to sedentary normal after eight months of nontraining.

Roskamm trained two groups of soldiers five days a week for four weeks. The results showed that both groups improved significantly during this period. A subsequent decrease in working capacity was found within two weeks after cessation of training for one of the two groups who refrained from training.

It is apparent from this review that training effects are both gained or lost rather quickly, and regular, continual stimulation is necessary in maintaining proper cardiorespiratory fitness.

MODE OF TRAINING   There are a multitude of training modes available. They vary from individual to group activities requiring varied levels of skill and being played under varying degrees of competitiveness. The question arises as to the relative value of these activities in producing cardiorespiratory fitness changes. Previous parts of this review have shown that certain quantities and combinations

TABLE 2.2. Effects of bed rest and subsequent training on cardio-vascular function of young men[a]

VARIABLE	UNITS	CONTROL	BED REST (20 days)	TRAINING (60 days)
Maximum oxygen uptake	ml/kg·min[b]	43.0	31.8	51.1
Maximum heart rate	beats/min	192.8	196.6	190.8
Maximum cardiac output	liters/min	20.0	14.8	22.8
Maximum stroke volume	ml	104.0	74.2	119.8
Heart volume	ml	860.0	770	895

[a]See reference number 73.
[b]Millimeters per kilogram of body weight per minute.

of intensity, duration, and frequency are necessary to produce and maintain a training effect.

Theoretically, in view of the results from the aforementioned training studies, it would appear that training effects would be independent of mode of activity if the various combinations of intensity, duration, and frequency are the same. Little evidence is available comparing the effects of various modes of training. With this in mind, we conducted a study to compare running, walking, and bicycling programs. In this study, frequency (three days per week), intensity (85 to 90 percent of maximum heart rate range), and duration (30 minutes) were held constant for a 20-week period. The results showed aerobic capacity (Figure 2.7) and other physiological variables to have similar improvements. Hence it appears that a variety of aerobic activities can be interchanged for improving and maintaining physical fitness.

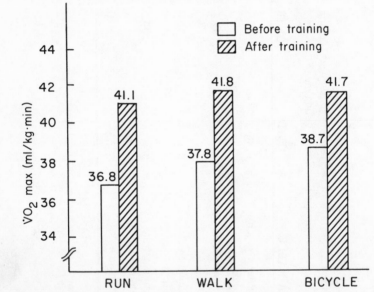

FIGURE 2.7. Effects of different modes of training on maximum oxygen uptake ($\dot{V}O_2$ max).

In general, moderate to high energy cost activities such as running (jogging), walking, swimming, bicycling, and many game-type activities show significant increases in cardiorespiratory fitness. In contrast, activities that are too intermittent and low in energy cost (below the intensity threshold) such as golf, bowling, and moderate calisthenics show no improvement. See Section 4 for more detailed information on the energy cost of various activities.

What about weight lifting? We often hear people complain about how tired they are after a weight training session. They also mention that their heart rate seems to be quite high after such a training program. Early studies testing the effect of weight training on cardiorespiratory fitness showed no significant improvement. Oftentimes, these programs emphasized heavy weights with long periods of rest between exercises. To better evaluate the effect of weight training on aerobic capacity, several studies have recently been conducted. In these experiments, men and women lifted moderate weights (approximately 50 to 60 percent of maximum) 10 to 15 times, on 8 to 12 exercises, using two to three sets (generally referred to as circuit weight training). The programs were kept as continuous as possible with little rest between exercises (15 to 30 seconds). The results from these regimens showed large increases in muscular strength but little (3 to 5%) or no change in aerobic capacity (see Figures 2.8 and 2.9). Therefore, weight training is not recommended as a program for improving cardiorespiratory fitness.

It should be noted that the heart rate—oxygen cost ratio is different for arm and leg work. For an equal heart rate, the oxygen cost of arm work is about 68 percent of that of leg work. Thus, the high heart rates found in some weight training activities may be misleading with regard to their energy cost value.

WEIGHT CONTROL

Obesity and overweight constitute two of the more significant medical and health problems in the United States today. The effects appear to be as much psychological as physiological. It has been estimated that as many as 10 million teenagers are overweight, representing approximately 20 percent of the total teenage population in the United States. As stated earlier, it has also been estimated that the average individual in this country who is 25 years of age or older will gain approximately 1 pound of additional weight per year. At the same time, the bone and muscle mass is decreasing by approximately 0.25 to 0.50 pound per year. This yields a net gain in fat of 1.25 to 1.50 pounds per year, 12.5 to 15 pounds in 10 years, or 37.5 to 45

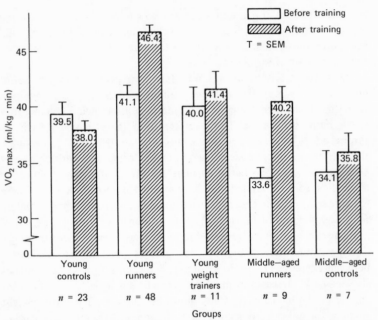

FIGURE 2.8. Effects of running and circuit weight training on maximum oxygen uptake ($\dot{V}O_2$ max).

pounds in 30 years. Again, this represents the *average* for our adult population.

OVERWEIGHT VERSUS OBESITY. Overweight was defined in Section 1 as exceeding the normal or standard weight for a specific height and frame size, when grouped by sex. In other words, if the average weight of the population as a whole for a particular height and frame size is found to be between 182 and 194 pounds, any weight in excess of 194 pounds would be considered overweight, and any weight below 182 pounds would be considered underweight, for any person of that height and frame size. Absolutely no consideration is given to the composition of that body weight. Individuals who are overweight might exceed the maximum allowable weight because they are carrying too much fat, or they may be of normal or below normal fat content, but have above average muscle development. Most football players fall into this last category. The term, overweight, in and of itself, is not necessarily undesirable nor does it imply serious medical concern. It

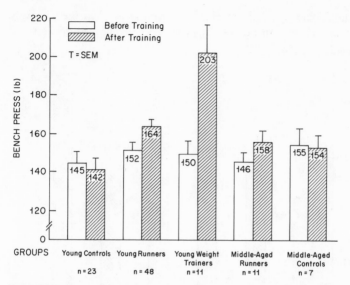

FIGURE 2.9. Effects of running (and moderate calisthenics exercises) and circuit weight training on one-repetition maximum bench press strength.

simply means that the individual has exceeded the population average for his or her height and frame size.

Obesity was previously defined as the condition where the individual is overfat, that is, one's total fat weight exceeds that considered optimal for the body weight. Normally, body fat is expressed in relative terms, where the fat weight is expressed as a percentage of the individual's total body weight. Although not specifically known or documented, the upper limit of ideal weight for men would include no more than 16 to 19 percent fat and for women, 22 to 25 percent fat. The standard for obesity would then be set at 25 percent fat for men and 30 to 35 percent fat for women.

Figures 2.10 and 2.11 show body weight and fat values of various groups of men. As mentioned in Section 1, body fat of women averages 5 to 10 percentage units higher than that of men. Marathon runners are not only lean but also light in body weight. Other athletic groups, such as football players, are relatively lean but are much heavier in body weight. As mentioned earlier, this extra weight would be mainly composed of lean body mass. In contrast, the sedentary middle-aged male or female is usually much heavier and fatter than the sedentary young person, and this extra weight would be composed of body fat.

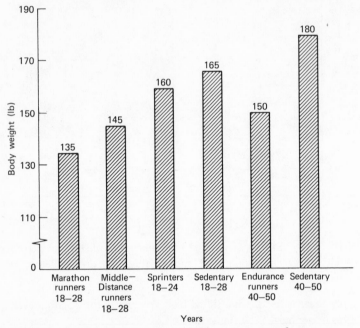

FIGURE 2.10. Body weight values of selected groups of men.

Health problems associated with obesity are far reaching. Respiratory problems are quite common among the obese. They have difficulty in normal breathing, a greater incidence of respiratory infections, and a lower exercise tolerance. Lethargy, associated with increased levels of carbon dioxide in the blood, and polycythemia (increased red blood cell production) because of lowered arterial blood oxygenation, are commonly found in obese persons. These can lead to blood clotting (thrombosis), enlargement of the heart, and congestive heart failure. Hypertension and atherosclerosis have also been linked to the obese individual, as have metabolic and endocrine disorders, such as impaired carbohydrate metabolism and diabetes. Obesity has also been associated with an increased risk of gallbladder disease, digestive diseases, and nephritis. More importantly, the mortality rate of the obese is substantially higher for each of these diseases than for people of normal weight. Few obese individuals are happy with their appearance and

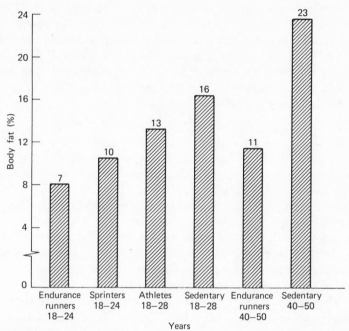

FIGURE 2.11. Percent body fat values of selected groups of men.

self-control and thus may be under continued stress and tension.

At one time, obesity was thought to be the result of basic hormonal imbalances in the blood, resulting from a malfunction of one or more of the endocrine, or hormone producing glands. At another time, obesity was considered to be the direct result of gluttony. Results of recent research, however, indicate that the causes of obesity are many and are often quite complex. A number of recent experimental studies on animals have established a link between obesity and heredity or genetic factors. Obesity has also been linked with physiological and psychological trauma. Hormonal imbalances, emotional trauma (anxiety and depression), and alterations in various mechanisms that regulate or control body stability have all been shown to be either directly or indirectly related to the onset of obesity. Environmental factors such as cultural habits, inadequate physical activity, and improper diets have also been shown to contribute to the problem of obesity. These last factors probably constitute the primary cause for the majority of the obese population. In fact, recent findings have shown that one's dietary or exercise habits early in life can affect later weight patterns. At present, the mechanism for the long-term influence is not well understood, but persons who are active as youngsters tend to develop fewer fat cells and their fat cell size is smaller. The tendency to have fewer and smaller fat cells is associated with less chance of becoming obese later in life. This emphasizes the need for good physical activity programs in pre-elementary and elementary school curricula.

ROLE OF EXERCISE IN WEIGHT CONTROL. What role does exercise play in the prevention, control, and treatment of obesity? For many years, it was a common belief that exercise was of little or no value in programs of weight reduction and control. Many examples were given demonstrating the tremendous number of hours of vigorous exercise necessary to obtain even small losses in body weight. Recent evidence shows, however, that physical inactivity is a major cause of obesity in the United States and may even be a far more significant factor than overeating. In addition, many studies have shown that substantial changes in body composition do result from an exercise program, even when diet remains unchanged.

When weight is lost by diet alone, a substantial amount of the total weight lost comes from the lean tissue, not fat tissue, and predominantly from the fluid spaces, that is, water loss. Most of the recent fad diets have emphasized low carbohydrate intake. This results in a depletion of the carbohydrate stored in the body. With a loss of 1 gram of carbohydrate, there is a concommitant loss of approximately 3 grams of water. From 3 to 5 pounds of weight loss per week can come from water loss associated with a loss of carbohydrate stored in the muscles and liver.

With exercise, there is typically a gain in lean body weight because of an increase in muscle mass (hypertrophy). In addition, there is a substantial loss in body fat. Typically, body weight changes little, if any, following the first six to eight weeks of an exercise program, since lean weight is increasing to about the same extent that fat weight is decreasing. The participant tends to be discouraged, since the bathroom scales show absolutely no or only modest progress. The body composition, however, has changed significantly, and that is the important consideration. The fact that the participant's clothes do not fit properly is the better indicator that positive change is occurring even though the actual weight lost is small.

When using exercise as a means for weight reduction, the total energy cost of the physical activity program is the most important consideration in designing a weight control program. Activities that are continuous in nature and have a moderate to high caloric expenditure such as running, walking, cycling, swimming, and vigorous game activities are recommended. Since there are approximately 3,500 calories in a pound of fat, it would require an expenditure of 3,500 calories to lose a pound of fat. By increasing caloric expenditure by 300 to 500 calories per day through a properly prescribed physical activity program, it would be possible to lose a pound of fat in 7 to 12 exercise sessions. For most people, this would mean a moderate jog for 30 minutes per day or a brisk walk for 45 to 60 minutes. If a *modest* diet was also followed, weight and fat reduction would occur at an even faster rate. Reducing food intake by one buttered slice of bread or one glass of dry white wine per day (approximately equivalent to 100 calories), combined with a 30-minute-per-day jogging program, 3 days per week (approximately equivalent to 0.2 to 0.3 pounds of weight loss per week), would result in a total weight loss of 20 to 30 pounds per year. Although this is only a one-half pound weight loss or less per week, patience does pay off, since this form of weight loss has been found to be more permanent.

Table 2.3 shows a comparison of body weight and fat changes resulting from training programs conducted with adult men and women 18 to 65 years of age. These data generally show reductions in body weight from 0 to 6.6 pounds and percent fat from 0 to 3.8 percent. Although changes of this magnitude are quite reasonable for estimated caloric expenditures encountered during these regimens, intergroup comparisons are difficult to make. The lack of dietary control and the quantifying and reporting of training data account for this difficulty.

Since changes in body weight and fat are related to the total energy expenditure of a program, the regimens that showed greater combinations of frequency, duration, or intensity tend to show greater change. The changes seem to manifest themselves with weeks of training, that is, programs of 8 to 10 weeks duration generally result in only small changes. It should be noted that with adult men and women the first few weeks of training are generally developmental in nature and do not necessarily have a high total energy output. Therefore, the shorter duration regimens may not allow enough time for full adaptation to occur. For example, in a jogging program, beginners will start by doing a combination of walking and jogging and slowly

TABLE 2.3. Comparison of body weight and percent fat changes with endurance training.

INVESTIGATOR	REFERENCE	SEX	AGE	n
Girandola	26	F	19	20
Smith	78	F	21	10
Golding	28	M	College+	4
Huibregtse	32	M	25	15
Brynteson	6	M	28	21
Pollock	57	M	32	11
Pollock	57	M	33	9
Wilmore	83	M	33	55
Wilmore	82	M	33	20
Wilmore	82	M	33	20
Pollock	[a]	M	35	9
Getchell	23	M	42	12
Getchell	23	F	35	11
Pollock	58	M	36	6
Pollock	58	M	37	5
Oscai	52	M	37	14
Misner	44	M	38	8
Pollock	62	M	38	26
Pollock	60	M	39	22
Ribisl	70	M	40	15
Terjung	80	M	40	15
Kilbom	36	M	41	42
Naughton	49	M	41	18
Skinner	76	M	42	15
Carter	10	M	47	7
Pollock	59	M	49	14
Myhre	48	M	53	10
Pollock	64	M	57	22

[a]Unpublished data, Institute for Aerobics Research, Dallas, Tex.
[b]Walk six miles per day at 3.0 miles per hour.

TABLE 2.3. Comparison of body weight and percent fat changes with endurance training. (Continued)

TRAINING (weeks)	TIME (min)	DAYS Per Week	ACTIVITY	CHANGE BODY WEIGHT (kg)	FAT (%)
10	7-15	3	Bike	+0.3	-0.4
7	16	3	Bike	+0.3	-0.7
25	—	4+	Run-cal.	-3.0	—
1-1/2	[b]	7	Walk	+0.6	—
5	30	5	Bike	-0.5	—
20	30	4	Run	-2.9	-1.0
20	30	2	Run	+0.1	+0.9
10	18	3	Run	-1.0	-1.1
10	12	3	Run	-0.6	—
10	24	3	Run	-1.4	—
20	30	3	Run	-1.7	-2.5
10	20	3	Run-walk	-0.8	—
10	20	3	Run-walk	-0.7	—
16	30	4	Run	-0.9	-3.3
16	30	2	Run	-0.8	+0.4
20	30	3	Run	-2.4	-2.2
8	30	3	Run	-0.8	-2.5
20	30	3	Run-walk-bike	-1.3	-1.8
20	45	2	Run	-0.7	-0.6
20	30	3	Run	-2.6	-0.7
6	12	5	Run in place	+0.5	-0.0
8-10	30	2+	Run	+0.3	—
28	30	3	Run	-2.1	—
24	35	3	Run-cal.	+0.1	-1.8
26	30	2+	Run	-3.0	-3.8
20	40	4	Walk	-1.3	-1.1
24	45	3	Run-games	-1.4	-3.1
20	30	3	Run-walk	-1.2	-1.6

progress to a continuous jog. Depending on age and initial level of fitness, it may take up to six months to be able to jog up to three continuous miles. Carter and Phillips found that middle-aged men who jogged for 30 minutes, three days per week for two years continued to lose body weight and fat for the first 12 months of the program. During the second year of training their body composition values leveled off and were maintained. Since their training regimen had not changed during the latter part of the first year and the second year, these results were not surprising. In order to lose more body weight and fat, the subjects would have had to increase their training load (caloric expenditure).

Another factor that makes the interpretation of training results difficult is the status of the participant's body composition. Persons who are obese tend to lose body weight and fat more readily than nonobese or lean individuals. Studies conducted on inmates showed little or no body weight or fat loss in high caloric expenditure programs. Inmates are generally on a reduced calorie diet after they enter prison and lose a substantial amount of body weight and fat. Their initial body fat values showed them to be 12 to 13 percent, which would be considered quite lean for men who averaged 27 years of age.

Is there a specific threshold of training (energy expenditure) that is necessary for weight reduction and fat loss? This is an interesting point, but difficult to quantify or speculate upon. Keeping in mind the many possible inconsistencies and confounding factors that are related to the results of studies using exercise as a means for weight control, we wish to speculate on existing evidence. It has been established that frequency, intensity, and duration of training, mode of activity, and initial level of fitness are important factors in formulating an exercise prescription. These factors relate to the total energy expenditure of the program and the rate at which a participant can tolerate endurance activity.

Cureton suggested that a minimum of 300 to 500 calories of energy expenditure was necessary to elicit optimal changes in cardiorespiratory fitness and body composition. Cooper, using a point system that is based upon oxygen expenditure, generally agrees with the 300 calorie threshold. These values coincide with jogging (running) regimens conducted for 20 to 30 minutes duration and walking programs of 40 to 60 minutes. The programs showing weight and fat reduction listed in Table 2.3 generally meet these requirements and those of less caloric cost show little or no change. One significant factor that influences the total caloric expenditure concept is frequency of training. Pollock and others have conducted four different two-day-per-week jogging studies in which the participants averaged from 600 to 1000 calories a week and showed no significant reductions in body weight or percent fat. This was somewhat perplexing considering that the number of miles trained and the calories expended per week were similar in two of the studies to three-day-per-week regimens that did show reductions. Although the rationale for this phenomenon is not clearly understood, it appears that two-day-per-week programs may not provide the continual stimulation necessary for a pronounced reduction in body fat.

Gwinup had obese women exercise daily for one year or longer with no dietary restrictions and found no weight loss until subjects' walk duration exceeded 30 minutes daily. Weight loss was directly related to time spent walking. Therefore, a minimal threshold for weight reduction and fat loss by endurance exercise alone would include the following: continuous physical activity of 20 to 30 minutes duration; exercise should be of sufficient intensity to expend 300 calories per exercise session; exercise frequency should be at least three-days per week; and, since total energy expenditure is highly related to weight and fat reduction, increased frequency, intensity, and duration of training should elicit greater reductions.

Weight training programs also have a significant effect on changing body composition but do not appear to reduce body weight. The changed composition results from an increase in lean body mass and fat loss. The final result would be a decrease in relative fat. Misner, using heavy weights in combination with fewer repetitions (three to eight), showed a larger increase in lean body mass than two other studies that used lighter weights and a higher number of repetitions (15 to 20). These findings showed the specificity of training and generally indicated that weight training with the proper combination of weight and repetitions is beneficial for increasing strength, losing fat and, at the same time, not building bulky muscles.

Several misconceptions have been accepted as fact over the years. First, it has been assumed that the obese individual eats more food than his or her lean counterpart. Several studies have shown just the opposite to be true, that is, the obese individual eats even less food. The major difference is that the obese individual is considerably more sedentary and expends far fewer calories each day. A second misconception that has existed for a number of years is that exercise, itself, stimulates the appetite to such an extent that voluntary food intake is increased as a result of exercise. This concept has also been proved to be incorrect when applied to moderate to strenuous endurance exercise. Studies have demonstrated that moderate to vigorous exercise of up to an hour in duration actually acts to depress the appetite. Thus, exercise does appear to be a mild appetite suppressant.

SPOT REDUCTION. The role of exercise in spot weight reduction is a controversial area. Many individuals, including athletes, believe that by exercising a specific area, the fat in that area will be selectively utilized, thus reducing the locally stored fat. Recent studies have shown the concept of spot reduction to be a myth, and they have shown that exercise, even when localized, draws from all of the fat stores of the body, not just from the local depots. A study by Gwinup and others demonstrated that the dominant arm of professional tennis players had greater muscular development than the nondominant arm because of the differences in activity levels of the two arms. No differences between arms were found in localized fat stores.

MUSCULAR STRENGTH AND ENDURANCE

Muscular strength refers to the absolute maximum amount of force that one can generate in an isolated movement of a single muscle or a group of muscles. The stronger the individual, the greater the force that he or she can generate. Muscular endurance refers to the ability to perform repeated contractions, as illustrated by the individual who attempts to perform as many sit-ups as possible in a 60-second period of time. Muscular endurance involves a specific muscle or group of muscles, whereas cardiorespiratory endurance involves the total body.

Strength and muscular endurance can be developed by any one, or a combination of three different modes or forms of training—isometric, isotonic, and isokinetic—using either eccentric (lenthening) or concentric (shortening) contractions. Isometric training involves exercising against a resistance greater than the force that can be applied, where there is no movement of the body parts. Pushing against a 20-story building results in a contraction of the involved muscles, but does not result in any perceptable movement of the body or the building. A whole series of isometric exercises have been devised that use parts of the body or common objects around the house as the source of resistance (see Figure 2.12). Isotonic training involves the actual movement or lifting of a constant resistance through the range of motion of the joint or joints involved. Lifting weights is a classic example of isotonic training. A constant resistance, that is, the weight, barbell, or dumbbell, is lfited theough the range of motion. Isokinetic training involves a constant speed of movement against a variable resistance. The strength of the muscle varies at different angles in the range of movement (see Figure 2.13), as a result of changes in the angle of pull and the respective leverage. Hence, when lifting a constant resistance, the muscle is not exercised to the same extent as it goes through the range of motion. With isokinetic training, the resistance changes to match the strength of the muscle at each point in the range of motion.This can be accomplished in one of several different ways, but it does require specialized equipment. With several of these devices, the rate of contraction is controlled at a set speed no matter how hard one pulls or pushes. Theoretically, this allows the maximal contraction of the muscle or muscles at each point in the entire range of motion.

STRENGTH TRAINING PROCEDURES. The concept of *isometric exercise* evolved in the early twentieth century, although it gained popularity and widespread support during the middle 1950s as a result of the work of two German investigators, Hettinger and Müeller. Their initial studies indicated that tremendous gains in strength resulted from isometric training procedures, and these gains were found to be greater than those resulting from the more traditional isotonic procedures. They claimed that isometric training would lead to increases of 5 percent of the original strength value per week as the result of a single six-second contraction per day, at only 67 percent of maximal contraction strength. Supposedly, little difference in improvement resulted when the tension was increased to 100 percent of maximal contraction strength, or when repeated exercises totalling 45 seconds were given.

Subsequent studies have been unable to totally confirm the original work by Hettinger and Müeller. Most of these studies have found substantial increases in strength with isometric training, but not of the magnatude claimed in the original studies. There has been support, however, for the contention that it does not require maximal con-

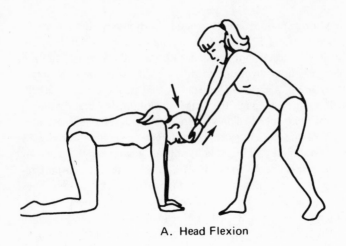

A. Head Flexion

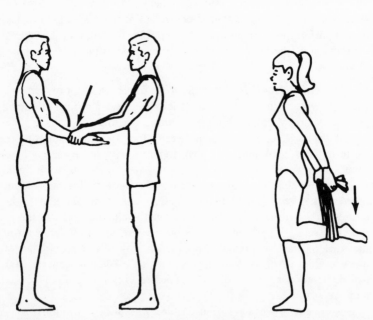

FIGURE 2.12. Illustration of an isometric contraction. (Courtesy of J. DiGennaro. *Individualized Exercise and Optimal Fitness: A Review Workbook for Men and Women.* Philadelphia: Lea & Fibeger, 1974, p. 41.)

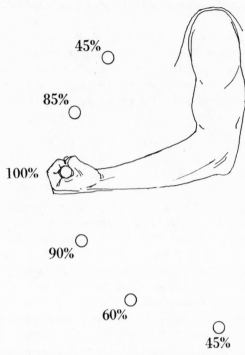

FIGURE 2.13. Variation in strength relative to the angle of contraction with 100 percent representing the angle where strength is maximal. (Courtesy of C.R. Jensen and A. G. Fisher. *Scientific Basis of Athletic Conditioning.* Philadelphia: Lea & Febiger, 1972, p. 76.)

traction or more than one 6-second contraction to attain significant gains in strength. One study compared two groups, one exercising at 67 percent of maximum contraction strength, one 6-second contraction per day, and the other at 80 percent of maximum contraction strength, five 6-second contractions per day. Both groups increased strength substantially, but the two groups did not differ with respect to the magnitude of the strength gains. This showed that one 6-second contraction per day was as effective for developing strength as contractions given more frequently and at higher levels of tension. More recent work by Müeller and Rohmert suggest that maximal contractions held for six-second periods, repeated 5 to 10 times per day, is a superior technique. Obviously, more research is necessary before any definite conclusions can be drawn relative to the most efficient way to gain strength through isometric exercise. There does appear to be good evidence to support the contention that isometric training should be conducted at several points in the full range of motion, since several studies have noted that the strength gain was specific to the angle of the joint at which the training was performed, that is, the strength gains were greatest at the angle where training was performed and decreased to very slight or no gains at other joint angles.

Isotonic training has traditionally involved the use of dumbbells, barbells, and weight pulleys. The system of progressive resistance exercise has been the preferred technique of isotonic training. As its name implies, progressive resistance exercise consists of gradually increasing the resistance against which a given muscle or muscle group must work, concomitant with the increase in strength, to progressively maintain a high relative muscle force or tension. DeLorme, and later work by DeLorme and Watkins, produced the initial efforts to systematize isotonic training through progressive resistance exercise techniques. Their system utilized heavy resistance and low repetitions to develop strength, power and volume of muscles, as opposed to light resistance and high repetitions to develop muscular endurance. Initially, it was suggested that the subject do 70 to 100 repetitions divided into 7 to 10 sets of 10 repetitions per set. Later, this was modified to the traditional DeLorme system in which three sets of 10 repetitions per set are performed. The 10-repetition maximum (10-RM) is determined as the greatest resistance that can be lifted ten, but no more than ten, consecutive times. The first set is performed at a resistance equal to 50 percent of 10-RM, the second at 75 percent of 10-RM, and the third at 100 percent of 10-RM. The resistance is increased periodically as strength increases. Several modifications of this system have been proposed, but they do not appear to offer any advantages over the system outlined above.

Many studies have looked at various combinations of sets and repetitions to optimize the training procedure. It would appear from an overview of all of these studies that isotonic weight training should be performed at 5- to 7-RM per set, performing three sets per training session to maximize strength gains. Training frequency should be three times per week, although this can be increased to five times per week if the muscles have been preconditioned to take this stress. The length of the total workout will be determined by the number of exercises performed and can vary from a few minutes to several hours. With longer workouts, specific exercises should be varied to alternate between upper limb, trunk, and lower limb exercises.

Isokinetic training procedures are relatively new in concept and practice. Introduced in 1968 by Perrine, the resistance is adjusted throughout the range of motion to match or accommodate the maximal possible force that can be applied by the muscles. Thus, if the individual is motivated to apply maximum force throughout the entire range of motion, the resistance will vary directly with the force to allow maximum performance throughout the same range. The concept of isokinetic training adds a new dimension to the area of strength training. With many isokinetic training devices, it is possible to vary the speed of contraction from very slow to extremely fast. Since there is a great deal of specificity to training, it is tempting to postulate that high-speed isokinetic training would provide the greatest stimulus for improvement in actual athletic performance, since athletic events are usually performed at high velocities. Preliminary research findings suggest that this is true.

COMPARISON OF ISOMETRIC, ISOTONIC, AND ISOKINETIC PROCEDURES. From the above discussions, it appears that each of the three strength training procedures produce substantial increases in strength, power, and muscular endurance. Does any one of the three offer a distinct advantage over the other two, or do all three provide equal gains in strength, power, and muscular endurance, for an equal quantity of time and effort invested? The majority of comparative studies conducted to-date have compared only isometric and isotonic procedures. This is because isokinetic training procedures were just recently introduced and are not widely accepted or understood. Clarke has recently summarized the results of those studies comparing isometric and isotonic procedures as follows.

1. Both isometric and isotonic procedures produce substantial gains in muscular strength. Although most studies indicated little, if any, difference between the two procedures, several studies have shown that isotonic exercise provides greater gains.

2. Muscular endurance is more effectively developed through isotonic procedures, and recovery from muscular fatigue is faster in muscles that have been trained isotonically. These results would be expected on the basis of the static nature of isometric exercise, where isotonic exercise is rhythmical and repetitive.

3. Isometric procedures appear to develop strength in only a limited portion of the total range of motion; therefore, isotonic procedures will produce a more uniform development of strength.

4. Isometric procedures can be used during a period of convalescence from injury. Normally, the injured limb is completely immobilized, and the subsequent lack of exercise will result in a reduction in both muscle size and strength. Isometric procedures involve no joint movements and can be safely and effectively used during the period of recovery from injury to prevent substantial loss of muscle size and function.

5. Isotonic procedures appear to cause a greater degree of muscle hypertrophy, which may or may not be a desired outcome of the muscle training program.

There are also several additional practical considerations that are important. Isometric exercises can be performed anywhere, at anytime, with little or no investment in equipment. On the negative side, there is literally no feedback as to how much improvement an individual experiences as he or she gains strength through isometric exercises. Individuals who lift weights get positive feedback when they increase the amount of weight on the bar as they become stronger. This lack of positive feedback with isometric exercise has led many individuals to abandon their isometric programs. Also, isometric exercises are potentially dangerous for older individuals and individuals who have diagnosed cardiovascular disease, such as coronary artery disease, hypertension, or those who have had strokes. When performing isometric exercises, it is typical for the individual to take in a deep breath, hold it, and then forcefully compress the air in the abdominal and thoracic cavities. This restricts the return of blood to the heart, increases blood pressure, and reduces the availability of blood to the heart muscle and brain.

As mentioned earlier, the research on isokinetic training is limited, since it represents a relatively new concept in strength training. A major advantage of isokinetic training over the more conventional types is in the area of rehabilitation. Isokinetic apparatus allow the muscle to exercise through a full range of motion with varying degrees of resistance. The resistance is dependant on the strength of the muscle at different angles in the range of motion. Several studies have shown isokinetic procedures to be as effective as isometric and isotonic training procedures in developing muscular strength and endurance. In a recent study, substantial differences were found between isokinetic and isotonic training procedures. Two groups training with isokinetic procedures, one at slow and one at fast limb speeds, and a third group training with isotonic procedures, trained three days per week for a total of eight weeks. Both isokinetic groups exhibited greater gains in strength and greater improvements in measurements of performance such as the 40-yard dash, softball throw for distance, and vertical jump. Considerably more research must be undertaken to provide greater insight into this new area of strength training.

FLEXIBILITY

Flexibility can be defined as the range of possible movement about a joint or a sequence of joints. As was mentioned in Section 1, in a study of several hundred adults who had complaints of chronic lower back problems, approximately 80 percent had muscle weakness and joint inflexibility diagnosed as the cause, while only 20 percent has a specific disease, lesion, or anatomical anomaly as the cause.

In a recent publication, Clarke summarized the research literature on flexibility and exercise as follows.

1. There is little agreement among researchers with regard to the definition and limits of "normal" flexibility, and what constitutes generally poor or exceptional flexibility.

2. Flexibility is highly specific to the individual joints, and measurements of flexibility in several body joints cannot be used to predict flexibility in other body joints.

3. Sufficient data are not yet available to generalize about the relationship of specific flexibility measures to sex and age.

4. Those connective tissues primarily responsible for resistance to movement include muscle, ligament, joint capsule, and tendon.

5. Insufficient data exist comparing the relative benefits of static versus ballistic stretching for improving joint mobility, although static stretching would seem to be a far safer and less stressful form of stretching. deVries has found this to result in the least possible reflex stimulation to the muscle or muscles being stretched.

6. Flexibility can be increased with exercise, but the magnitude of increase and the joints affected depend totally on the type or form of exercise, that is, change is specific to the activity.

Leighton reported a series of studies on college and champion male athletes in the sports of baseball, basketball, gymnastics, swimming, track, weight lifting, and wrestling. He used a specific device to measure the full range of joint mobility in 30 different joint movements (Flexometer). The values for a randomly selected group of 16-year-old boys were used for comparative purposes. The swimmers and baseball players showed the highest degree of flexibility, exceeding the 16-year-old boys' comparative group on 20 of the 30 joint movements. Basketball players exceeded the comparative group on 14 of the joint movements, were lower on eight, and were the same on eight. Shot and discus throwers, and gymnasts were higher on 15, lower on 6, and the same on 9 joint movements. Wrestlers had the poorest flexibility of all groups, exceeding the comparative groups on only eight joint movements. It was concluded that the unique movement patterns of each sport influence to a great extent the degree of flexibility gained by the athletes participating in these various sports.

At one time, it was felt that weight training would cause greatly enlarged muscles, which would, in turn, reduce joint flexibility. Studies have not supported this contention. Weight lifters and body builders who achieved international recognition for their lifting accomplishments and physiques were found to have greater flexibility than the normal population. Other studies have shown increases in flexibility resulting from weight training programs, provided that the weight training was performed throughout the full range of joint motion, that is, these athletes generally practice flexibility exercises along with their normal routine.

Finally, stretching exercises, designed specifically for increasing joint mobility or flexibility, have been shown to produce the most significant improvement. An entire series of stretching exercises is provided in Section 4. Adherence to the stretching routine for a period of only several weeks will result in a remarkable improvement in joint flexibility.

SUMMARY

Research findings showed that improvement in cardiorespiratory endurance and reduction in body weight and fat were dependent on the intensity, duration, and frequency of the training program. Intensity and duration of training were found to be interrelated with the total calories expended being the important factor. Although there appears to be a minimal threshold for improving cardiorespiratory fitness (50 to 60% of maximum), generally programs of 20 to 40 minutes of continuous activity, performed three to five days per week, showed significant improvement in fitness and weight control. The advantages of exercise as a means of weight control were also discussed. Recent studies showed that the concept of spot reduction was not valid. Exercise would draw energy from all fat stores in the body, not just the ones from the area being exercised.

The three basic types of strength training were discussed: isometric, isotonic, and isokinetic. It was shown that all three systems of exercise were effective in developing muscular strength. The advantages and disadvantages of each system were discussed.

The last portion of the section defines flexibility and discusses its importance in health and fitness. In general, flexibility is lost rather quickly if special exercises are not practiced on a regular basis.

REFERENCES

1. Allen, T.E., R.J. Byrd, and D.P. Smith. "Hemodynamic consequences of circuit weight training." *Res. Q., 43*:299-306 (1976).

2. Åstrand, P.O., and B. Saltin. "Maximal oxygen uptake and heart rate in various types of muscular activity." *J. Appl. Physiol., 16*:977-981 (1961).

3. Åstrand, P.O., and K. Rodahl. *Textbook of Work Physiology*, 2nd Ed., New York: McGraw-Hill, 1977.

4. Balke, B., and R. Ware. "An experimental study of physical fitness of air force personnel." *US Armed Forces Med. J., 10*:675-688 (1959).

5. Boileau, R.A., E.R. Buskirk, D.H. Horstman, J. Mendez, and W.C. Nicholas. "Body composition changes in obese and lean men during physical conditioning." *Med. Sci. Sports, 3*:183-189 (1971).

6. Brynteson, P., and W.E. Sinning "The effects of training frequencies on the retension of cardiovascular fitness." *Med. Sci. Sports, 5*:29-33 (1973).

7. Burke, E.J., and B.D. Franks. "Changes in $\dot{V}O_2$ max resulting from bicycle training at different intensities holding total mechanical work constant." *Res. Q., 46*:31-37 (1975).

8. Cooper, K.H. *The New Aerobics.* New York: J.B. Lippincott, 1970.

9. Costill, D.L., and E. Winrow. "Maximal oxygen intake among marathon runners." *Arch. Phys. Med. Rehabil., 51*:317-320 (1970).

10. Carter, J.E.L., and W.H. Phillips. "Structural changes in exercising middle-aged males during a 2-year period." *J. Appl. Physiol., 27*:787-794 (1969).

11. Clarke, D.H. "Adaptations in strength and muscular endurance resulting from exercise." In: *Exercise and Sport Sciences Review,* Jack H. Wilmore (ed.). Vol. I, New York: Academic Press, 1973.

12. Clarke, H.H. "Development of muscular strength and endurance." *Physical Fitness Research Digest.* President's Council on Physical Fitness and Sports, Series 4, No. 1, January 1974.

13. Clarke, H.H. "Joint and body range of movement." *Physical Fitness Research Digest.* President's Council on Physical Fitness and Sports. Washington, D.C., Series 5, No. 4, October 1975.

14. Charney, H.C., M. Goodman, M. McBride, B. Lyon, and R. Pratt. "Childhood antecedents of adult obesity." *New England J. Med., 295*:6-9 (1976).

15. Cureton, T.K., and E.E. Phillips. "Physical fitness changes in middle-aged men attributable to equal eight-week periods of training, nontraining and retraining." *J. Sports Med. Phys. Fitness, 4*:1-7 (1964).

16. Cureton, T.K. *The Physiological Effects of Exercise Programs upon Adults.* Springfield, Ill.: C.C. Thomas, 1969.

17. Davies, C.T.M., and A.V. Knibbs. "The training stimulus, the effects of intensity, duration and frequency of effort on maximum aerobic power output." *Int. Z. Angew. Physiol., 29*:299-305 (1971).

18. DeLorme, T.L. "Restoration of muscle power by heavy resistance exercise." *J. Bone and Joint Surgery, 27*:645-667 (1945).

19. DeLorme, T.L., and A.L. Watkins. "Techniques of progressive resistance exercise." *Arch. Phys. Med., 29*:263-273 (1948).

20. deVries, H.A. *Physiology of Exercise for Physical Education*

and Athletics. 2nd Ed. Dubuque, Ia.: W.C. Brown, 1974.

21. Drinkwater, B.L., S.M. Horvath, and C.L. Wells. "Aerobic power of females, ages 10 to 68." *J. Geront., 30*:385-394 (1975).

22. Fox, S.M., J.P. Naughton, and W.L. Haskell. "Physical activity and the prevention of coronary heart disease." *Ann. Clin. Res., 3*: 404-432 (1971).

23. Getchell, L.H., and J.C. Moore. "Physical training: comparative responses of middle-aged adults." *Arch. Phys. Med. Rehabil., 56*:250-254 (1975).

24. Gettman, L.R., M.L. Pollock, J.L. Durstine, A. Ward, J. Ayres, and A.C. Linnerud. "Physiological responses of men to 1, 3, and 5 day per week training programs." *Res. Q., 47*:638-646 (1976).

25. Gettman, L.R., J. Ayres, M.L. Pollock, L. Durstine, and W. Grantham. "Physiological effects of circuit strength training and jogging on adult men." Submitted for publication, 1977.

26. Girandola, R.N. "Body composition changes in women: Effects of high and low exercise intensity." *Arch. Phys. Med. Rehab., 57*:297-300 (1976).

27. Gledhill, N., and R.B. Eynon. "The intensity of training." In: *Training Scientific Basis and Application.* Taylor, A.W., Howell, M.L. (eds.). Springfield, Ill.: C.C. Thomas, 1972, pp. 97-102.

28. Golding, L. "Effects of physical training upon total serum cholesterol levels." *Res. Q., 32*:499-505 (1961).

29. Gwinup, G. "Effect of exercise alone on the weight of obese women." *Arch. Int. Med., 135*:676-680 (1975).

30. Hill, J.S. "The effects of frequency of exercise on cardiorespiratory fitness of adult men." M.S. Thesis, University of Western Ontario, London, 1969.

31. Hollmann, W., and H. Venrath. "Experimentelle untersuchungen zur bedeutung aines trainings unterhalb and oberhalb der dauerbeltz stungsgranze." In: *Carl Diem Festschrift,* Korbs (ed.). W. u. a. Frankfurt/Wein, 1962.

32. Huibregtse, W.H., H.H. Hartley, L.R. Jones, W.D. Doolittle, and T.L. Criblez. "Improvement of aerobic work capacity following

nonstrenuous exercise." *Arch. Environ. Health, 27*:12-15 (1973).

33. Karvonen, M., K. Kentala, and O. Muslala. "The effects of training heart rate: a longitudinal study." *Ann. Med. Exptl. Biol. Fenn., 35*:307-315 (1957).

34. Kasch, F.W., and J.L. Boyer. "Exercise therapy in hypertensive men." *JAMA, 211*:1668-1671 (1970).

35. Kendrick, Z.B., M.L. Pollock, T.N. Hickman, and H.S. Miller. "Effects of training and detraining on cardiovascular efficiency." *Amer. Corr. Ther. J., 25*:79-83 (1971).

36. Kilbom, A., L. Hartley, B. Saltin, J. Bjure, G. Grimby, and I. Åstrand. "Physical training in sedentary middle-aged and older men." *Int. Scand. J. Clin. Lab. Invest., 24*:315-322 (1969).

37. Klissouras, V. "Heritability of adaptive variation." *J. Appl. Physiol., 31*:338-344 (1971).

38. Knuttgen, H.G., L.O. Nordesjo, B. Ollander, and B. Saltin. "Physical conditioning through interval training with young male adults." *Med. Sci. Sports, 5*:220-226 (1973).

39. Kraus, H., and W. Raab, *Hypokinetic Disease.* Springfield, Ill.: C.C. Thomas, 1961.

40. Leighton, J.R. "Flexibility characteristics of four specialized skill groups of college athletes." *Arch. Phys. Mental Rehab., 38*: 24 (1957).

41. Leighton, J.R. "Flexibility characteristics of three specialized skill groups of champion athletes." *Arch. Phys. Mental Rehab., 38*: 580 (1957).

42. Mayhew, J.L., and P.M. Gross. "Body composition changes in young women with high resistance weight training." *Res. Q., 45*:433-439 (1974).

43. Milesis, C.A., M.L. Pollock, M.D. Bah, J.J. Ayres, A. Ward, and A.C. Linnerud. "Effects of different durations of training on cardiorespiratory function, body composition and serum lipids." *Res. Q., 47*:716-725 (1976).

44. Misner, J.E., R.A. Boileau, B.H. Massey, and J.H. Mayhew. "Alterations in body composition of adult men during selected

physical training programs." *J. Amer. Geriatr. Soc. 22*:33-38 (1974).

45. Mitchell, J., B. Sproule, and C. Chapman. "The physiological meaning of the maximal oxygen intake test." *J. Clin. Invest., 37*: 538-547 (1958).

46. Moody, D.L., J. Kollias, and E.R. Buskirk. "The effect of a moderate exercise program on body weight and skinfold thickness in overweight college women." *Med. Sci. Sports., 1*:75-80 (1969).

47. Mueller, E.A., and W. Rohmert. "Die geschwindigkeit der muskelkraft zunahme bei isometrischen training." *Intern. Zeitschrift Angewandte Physiol., 19*:403-419 (1963).

48. Myhre, L., S. Robinson, A. Brown, and F. Pyke. Changes observed in pulmonary function of old men following six months of physical training. Paper presented to the American College of Sports Medicine, Albuquerque, New Mexico, 1970.

49. Naughton, J., and F. Nagle. "Peak oxygen intake during physical fitness program for middle-aged men." *JAMA, 191*:899-901 (1965).

50. Naughton, J., and H.K. Hellerstein. *Exercise Testing and Exercise Training in Coronary Heart Disease.* New York: Academic Press, 1973.

51. Olree, H.D., B. Corbin, J. Penrod, and C. Smith. "Methods of achieving and maintaining physical fitness for prolonged space flight." Final Progress Report to NASA, Grant No. NGR-04-002-004, 1969.

52. Oscai, L.B., T. Williams, and B. Hertig. "Effects of exercise on blood volume." *J. Appl. Physiol., 24*:622-624 (1968).

53. Oscai, L.B. "The role of exercise in weight control." In: *Exercise and Sport Sciences Reviews,* J.H. Wilmore (ed.), Vol. 1. New York: Academic Press, 1973, pp. 103-125.

54. Oscai, L.B., S.P. Babirak, F.B. Dubach, J.A. McGarr, and C.N. Spirakis. "Exercise or food restriction: Effect on adipose tissue cellularity." *Amer. J. Physiol., 227*:901-904 (1974).

55. Perrine, J.J. "Isokinetic exercise and the mechanical energy potentials of muscle." *J. Health Phys. Ed. Red., 39*:40-44 (1968).

56. Pipes, T.V., and J.H. Wilmore, "Isokinetic vs. isotonic strength training in adult men." *Med. Sci. Sports 7*:262-274 (1975).

57. Pollock, M.L., T.K. Cureton, and L. Greninger. "Effects of frequency of training on working capacity, cardiovascular function, and body composition of adult men." *Med. Sci. Sports, 1*:70-74 (1969).

58. Pollock, M.L., J. Tiffany, L. Gettman, R. Janeway, and H. Lofland. "Effects of frequency of training on serum lipids, cardiovascular function, and body composition." In: *Exercise and Fitness,* B.D. Franks (ed.). Chicago: Athletic Institute, 1969, pp. 161-178.

59. Pollock, M.L., H. Miller, R. Janeway, A.C. Linnerud, B. Robertson, and R. Valentino. "Effects of walking on body composition and cardiovascular function of middle-aged men." *J. Appl. Physiol., 30*:126-130 (1971).

60. Pollock, M.L., J. Broida, Z. Kendrick, H.S. Miller, R. Janeway, and A.C. Linnerud, "Effects of training two days per week at different intensitites on middle-aged men." *Med. Sci. Sports, 4*: 192-197 (1972).

61. Pollock, M.L. "The quantification of endurance training programs." In: *Exercise and Sport Sciences Reviews,* J.H. Wilmore, (ed.). *Vol. I,* New York: Academic Press, 1973, pp. 155-188.

62. Pollock, M.L., J. Dimmick, H.S. Miller, Z. Kendrick, and A.C. Linnerud. "Effects of mode of training on cardiovascular function and body composition of middle-aged men." *Med. Sci. Sports, 7*:139-145 (1975).

63. Pollock, M.L., E.E. Laughridge, B. Coleman, A.C. Linnerud, and A. Jackson. "Prediction of body density in young and middle-aged women." *J. Appl. Physiol., 38*:745-749 (1975).

64. Pollock, M.L., G.A. Dawson, H.S. Miller, Jr., A. Ward, D. Cooper, W. Headley, A.C. Linnerud, and M.M. Nomeir. "Physiologic response of men 49 to 65 years of age to endurance training."

J. Amer. Geriatr. Soc., *24*:97-104 (1976).

65. Pollock, M.L., T. Hickman, Z. Kendrick, A. Jackson, A.C. Linnerud, and G. Dawson. "Prediction of body density in young and middle-aged men." *J. Appl. Physiol.*, *40*:300-304 (1976).

66. Pollock, M.L., A. Jackson, J. Ayres, A. Ward, A.C. Linnerud, and L.R. Gettman. "Body composition of elite class distance runners." *Ann. NY Acad. Sci.* 301: 361-370 (1977).

67. Pollock, M.L., and A. Jackson. "Body composition: Measurement and changes resulting from physical training." Proceedings 1977 Annual Meeting of the National College Physical Education Association for Men and the National Association of Physical Education for College Women, Orlando, FL, 1977.

68. Pollock, M.L. "Submaximal and maximal working capacity of elite distance runners—Part I. Cardiorespiratory aspects." *Ann. NY Acad. Sci. 301*:310-322 (1977).

69. Rarick, G.L., and G.L. Larsen. "Observations on frequency and intensity of isometric muscular effort in developing static muscular strength in post-pubescent males." *Res. Q.*, *29*:333-341 (1958).

70. Ribisl, P.M. "Effects of training upon the maximal oxygen uptake of middle-aged men." *Int. Z. Angew. Physiol.*, *26*:272-278 (1969).

71. Roskamm. H. "Optimum patterns of exercise for healthy adults." *Canad. Med. Ass. J.*, *96*:895-899 (1967).

72. Saltin, B., and P.O. Åstrand. "Maximal oxygen uptake in athletes." *J. Appl. Physiol.*, *23*:353-358 (1967).

73. Saltin B., G. Blomqvist, J. Mitchell, R.L. Johnson, K. Wildenthal, and C.B. Chapman. "Response to exercise after bed rest and after training." *Circulation, 37* and *38,* Suppl. 7, 1-78 (1968).

74. Saltin, B., L. Hartley, A. Kilbom, and I. Åstrand. "Physical training in sedentary middle-aged and older men." *Scand. J. Clin. Lab. Invest.*, *24*:323-334 (1969).

75. Shephard, R.J. "Intensity, duration and frequency of exercise as determinants of the response to a training regime." *Int. Z. Angew. Physiol.*, *26*:272-278 (1969).

76. Skinner, J., J. Holloszy, and T. Cureton. "Effects of a program of endurance exercise on physical work capacity and anthropometric measurements of fifteen middle-aged men." *Amer. J. Cardiol.*, *14*:747-752 (1964).

77. Skinner, J. "The cardiovascular system with aging and exercise." In: *Physical Activity and Aging.* D. Brunner, and E. Jokl (eds). Baltimore: University Park Press, 1970, pp. 100-108.

78. Smith, D.P., and F.W. Stransky. "The effect of training and detraining on the body composition and cardiovascular response of young women to exercise." *J. Sports Med.*, *16*:112-120 (1976).

79. Taylor, H.E., E. Buskirk, and A. Henschel. "Maximal oxygen intake as an objective measure of cardio-respiratory performance." *J. Appl. Physiol.*, *8*:77-80 (1955).

80. Terjung, R.L., K.M. Baldwin, J. Cooksey, B. Samson, and R.A. Sutter. "Cardiovascular adaptation to twelve minutes of mild daily exercise in middle-aged sedentary men." *J. Amer. Geriatr. Soc.*, *21*:164-168 (1973).

81. U.S. Department of Health, Education and Welfare, Public Health Service. *Obesity and Health.* Washington, D.C.: Government Printing Office, 1966.

82. Wilmore, J.H., J. Royce, R.N. Girandola, F.I, Katch, and V.L. Katch. "Physiological alterations resulting from a 10-week program of jogging." *Med. Sci. Sports, 2:* 17-14 (1970).

83. Wilmore, J.H., J. Royce, R.N. Girandola, F.I. Katch, and V.L. Katch. "Body composition changes with a 10-week jogging program." *Med. Sci. Sports, 2*:113-117 (1970).

84. Wilmore, J.H., and W.L. Haskell. "Body composition and endurance capacity of professional football players." *J. Appl. Physiol.*, *33*:564-567 (1972).

85. Wilmore, J.H. "Inferiority of female athletes: myth or reality." *J. Sports Med.*, *3*:1-6 (1975).

86. Wilmore, J.H. *Athletic Training and Physical Fitness: Physiological Principles and Practices of the Conditioning Process.* Boston: Allyn and Bacon, 1977.

87. Wilmore, J.H. R.B. Parr, P.A. Vodak, T.J. Barstow, T.V. Pipes,

P. Ward, and P. Leslie. "Strength, endurance, BMR, and body composition changes with circuit weight training." (Abstract) *Med. Sci. Sports,* 8:58-60 (1976).

88. Wilson, Nancy L. (ed.). *Obesity.* Philadelphia: F.A. Davis, 1969.

Section 3
Medical Screening and Evaluation Procedures

PRELIMINARY CONSIDERATIONS

In the evaluation process, we are concerned with obtaining certain preliminary information about the person being evaluated, such as a personal medical history, as well as the administration of a comprehensive battery of tests. The purpose of having this information is to provide the physician, and/or program director and exercise leader with sufficient information so that an accurate and safe exercise program can be prescribed.

Preliminary information should include such items as a physical examination and/or consultation with the family physician, completion of a medical history questionnaire and its discussion, explanation and signing of an informed consent form, and if possible, an exercise tolerance test during which the electrocardiogram (ECG) and blood pressure are monitored. The medical history form should include a record of personal and family history of coronary heart disease and the associated risk factors, present medication and treatment, eating habits and diet analysis, smoking history, and current physical activity pattern. Also, any other pertinent medical problems and physical disabilities should be listed. Thus, the information obtained in the preliminary evaluation should help to identify in advance the person who might be classified as a high risk for testing and program participation.

The informed consent form should provide the participant with an adequate understanding of the tests and program, and the potential risks that may be involved. In this way, individuals should know exactly what they are getting into prior to being tested and becoming a participant in an exercise program. All testing information should be held in strict confidence and not be released to anyone without permission. Also, participants should not be forced, coerced, or inadequately advised with the objective of obtaining a better performance on a test or increasing adherence to a program. Such a procedure is unethical, violates human rights, and is against policy established by the federal government and most professional organizations. See Appendix A, Tables A.1 and A.2 for an example of an informed consent form and medical history questionnaire. Also, refer to publications provided by the American College of Sports Medicine and the American Heart Association (see references 1 to 3).

Is it important to have a physical examination and take tests before starting an exercise program? The answer is yes to both questions, although there is some flexibility in the requirements, dependent upon the participant's age, status of health, family history, and present fitness level. If possible, it would be desirable for all persons to have a complete physical examination including a 12-lead resting and exercise ECG prior to their physical fitness evaluation. As mentioned earlier, the more information known about a participant before training, the safer and more accurate the exercise prescription. If a person is under 35 years of age and considered a low risk for coronary heart disease, the requirements can be less stringent.

What is meant by low- and high-risk individuals? The term "at risk" is associated with a person's risk for having coronary heart disease. A low-risk person would be asymptomatic (no chest discomfort, shortness of breath, etc.) and under 35 years of age, with no previous history of coronary heart disease or no known primary risk factors that are associated with it (high blood pressure, elevated blood fats and sugar, smoking, obesity, family history, "A" type behavior pattern, and abnormal ECG findings). For persons over 35 years of age, and/or who are symptomatic to coronary heart disease, or have known risk factors for it, a medical examination including a resting and exercise ECG are strongly recommended.

To rate one's risk for developing coronary heart disease, see Table 3.1. Also see Tables A.4 to A.13, Appendix A, for age- and sex-adjusted norms for many of these measures. Listed are the major risk factors that are associated with developing coronary heart disease. At the present time, the relative values for each risk are only arbitrary and will take many more years of study to evaluate precisely. In the mean time, the values presented in Table 3.1 can be considered the best estimates from the literature at the present time. A very important point to remember is that being at a high risk in more than one factor greatly increases one's chance of developing heart disease. For example, the chances of developing coronary heart disease jumps from onefold to nearly fourfold when a person goes from having one to three primary factors (see Figure 1.3). For the purpose of rating potential risk, having two or less factors puts one in a low-risk category, while three to four factors and above puts one in the moderate- and high-risk categories, respectively.

Although most people can be safely evaluated and placed into an exercise program, under certain conditions it might be recommended that certain individuals not exercise. Conditions contraindicative to exercise would include congestive heart failure, acute heart attack, acute infectious disease, severe valvular problems (heart), dangerous rhythm problems of the heart, severe angina (chest discomfort) with and without effort, and active myocarditis. There are also other medical conditions that are considered of a less stringent nature, but still put the participant in a position whereby special precautions during exercise testing and exercise prescription should be taken. For more detailed information concerning these conditions, see reference numbers 1 to 3, 17, 26, and 37.

Thus far, we have discussed the desirability of having certain preliminary information and a medical examination prior to entering an exercise program. In addition to medical screening, a thorough physical fitness evaluation is also recommended. Although there is some duplication in classifying tests, the main difference between a medical screening test and a physical fitness test is: (1) a medical test classifies a person as to health and disease status, and provides an estimation of one's risk of developing coronary heart disease; and (2) a physical

TABLE 3.1. Risk of developing coronary heart disease

RISK FACTOR	VERY LOW	RELATIVE LEVEL OF RISK			
		LOW	MODERATE	HIGH	VERY HIGH
Blood pressure (mmHg)					
Systolic	<110	120	130-140	150-160	170>
Diastolic	< 70	76	82-88	94-100	106>
Cigarettes (per day)	Never None in 1 yr	5	10-20	30-40	50>
Cholesterol (mm/100 cc)	<180	200	220-240	260-280	300>
Triglycerides (mm/100 cc)	< 80	100	150	200	300>
Glucose (mg/100 cc)	< 80	90	100-110	120-130	140>
Body fat (%)					
Men	< 12	16	22	25	30>
Women	< 15	20	25	33	40>
Stress-Tension	Almost never	Occasional	Frequent	Nearly constant	

Physical activity minutes above 6 Cal/min (5 METS)[a] per week	240	180-120	100	80-60	30<
ECG stress test abnormality (ST depression-mm) [b]	0	0	0.5	1	2>
Family history of premature heart attack[c] (blood relative)	0	1	2	3	4>
Age	< 30	35	40	50	60>

[a] A MET is equal to the oxygen cost at rest. One MET is generally equal to 3.5 milliliters per kilogram of body weight per minute of oxygen uptake or 1.2 calories per minute.
[b] Other ECG abnormalities are also potentially dangerous and are not listed here.
[c] Premature heart attack refers to <60 years of age.

TABLE 3.2. Recommended testing program for adults

FITNESS CATEGORY	PLAN A[a]
Cardiorespiratory Rest Exercise	Heart rate, blood pressure, ECG Stress test to functional maximum with heart rate, blood pressure, and ECG monitoring
Body composition	Percent fat by underwater weighing or equivalent, skinfold and girth measures, height and weight Determine ideal weight
Blood measures	Serum cholesterol, triglycerides, glucose, high- and low-density lipoprotein
Strength[d]	One-repetition bench press
Muscular endurance[d]	All-out pushups, bent leg sit-ups for one minute
Flexibility	Sit and reach

[a]Most preferred plan of testing physical fitness and risk factors for coronary heart disease.
[b]Next most preferred plan of testing.
[c]Least preferred plan of testing.
[d]Not appropriate for hypertensive and high-risk individual.
[e]Plan C, cardiorespiratory, should not be used for diagnostic purposes. Persons over 35 years of age or at high risk should have an ECG monitored, exercise tolerance test first.

PLAN B[b]	PLAN C[ce]
Same	Heart rate, blood pressure
Submaximal test with heart rate, blood pressure, and ECG monitoring	Submaximal test without ECG and blood pressure monitoring, and maximal field-type tests
Percent fat by skinfold and girth measures, height and weight	Percent fat by weight and girth, height
Same	Same
Serum cholesterol, triglycerides, and glucose	Serum cholesterol
Same	Same
Same	Same
Same	Same

fitness evaluation classifies a person as to status of fitness. The results from both the medical and fitness tests are also used as a basis for exercise prescription and a baseline for future comparisons. Like the medical examination, there can be some flexibility in the testing program, dependent upon one's health status, age, present fitness and activity level, and risk for coronary heart disease. Table 3.2 lists the major categories of fitness and the test items that will be discussed. Although the physical fitness evaluation can be thought of in broader terms, we feel that these categories and test items are sufficient for the basic needs of the adult population.

The test items listed in Table 3.2 become less complex and expensive as we go from plan A to plan C. In some cases the level of accuracy and diagnostic capability of the tests are also less between plans. The exercise tests listed under Plan C, cardiorespiratory, should not be used as a diagnostic test. Persons over 35 years of age or at high risk should take an ECG monitored exercise tolerance test prior to taking a fitness test listed under Plan C, cardiorespiratory. Medical advisors and program directors, as well as the participants, should take the cost, risk, and feasibility aspects of testing into consideration before setting up a test battery. Except for the blood measures, each aspect of testing listed in Table 3.2 will be discussed in the following sections, or in Appendix A.

The *blood serum measures* listed in Table 3.2 are standard procedures and can be determined rather easily and economically by most medical laboratories. The blood sample should be drawn at least 12 to 14 hours after the last meal, and a person should have refrained from exercise and alcohol consumption for at least 24 hours. The determination of high- and low-density lipoproteins gives a more accurate assessment of blood fats, but is expensive. To complete the risk factor profile shown in Table 3.1, the determination of serum cholesterol, triglycerides, and glucose is necessary.

EVALUATION PROCEDURES

INITIAL EVALUATION. The medical and fitness evaluations are used as a basis for exercise prescription. The results of the initial tests are used as a baseline for future comparisons. With respect to the latter statement, tests are excellent motivators for the participants in that they provide objective evidence as to their initial status (health and fitness), as well as the progress and benefits attained from a regular exercise program. To the contrary, if one is irregular or not putting in sufficient time and effort in to training, then it may give added motivation to better follow or to change the exercise prescription.

For the first evaluation many persons are apprehensive and thus may not do as well on some test items. Apprehension will adversely affect most of the resting and submaximal cariorespiratory tests. For example, heart rate would be greatly elevated under these conditions. Many tests are sensitive to time of day and whether one has eaten or smoked just prior to testing. Individuals usually improve their performance on a maximal exercise test with some practice. In many cases it would improve the test results if participants had a chance to practice the tests and become familiar with the laboratory setting (habituation) before initial testing. If a tester cannot use ideal conditions (fasting, time of day) for testing, then the conditions in which the tests are administered should be noted and standardized for future comparisons.

Heart rate is particularly susceptible to time of day, smoking, apprehension, coffee (and other stimulants), food, tension, temperature, and so on. Therefore, it is particularly important to standardize conditions for resting and submaximal heart rate tests. Maximal heart rate is not generally affected like resting and submaximal exercise values. Most cardiorespiratory tests should have a minimum of three hours of controlled conditions prior to testing. For more details on the standardization and interpretation of submaximal and maximal tests refer to the work of Taylor et al (see references 33 and 35).

FOLLOW-UP EVALUATIONS. How often should follow-up examinations be administered? Unless something unusual is found in one's initial tests, an interval history and physical examination are recommended every two years for persons under 35 years of age, approximately every 18 months between 35 and 40, and yearly after 40 years of age. Under normal circumstances a physical fitness test battery should be administered after approximately three to six months and again after one year of training. Yearly fitness evaluations are recommended after the first year.

Although fitness takes many months to attain, a progress check at three to six months is important for evaluating the participant's progress. With this information the participant's exercise prescription can be verified and modified as necessary. Not only does the progress check give the physician and program director vital information as to how the participant is getting along in the program but also it acts as a motivational tool to the participant. Many times a waning interest occurs about 10 to 15 weeks after beginning training, and therefore a motivational lift can help at this stage.

CARDIORESPIRATORY FITNESS. Many people who become interested in beginning a personal physical fitness program ask what tests should be taken prior to starting the program? They understand the idea behind the recommended testing program outlined in Table 3.2, but wonder if there is anything else they can do at home to evaluate their fitness level. This is a good question and here we provide the participant with more specific recommendations on tests and evaluation procedures.

The recommendation for a maximal exercise tolerance test to determine functional capacity was stated earlier. This was established as the most valid means of assessing cardiorespiratory fitness (Plan A, Table 3.2). Monitored submaximal (Plan B) and unmonitored submaximal and field tests (Plan C) are considered less accurate. Also, in the case of the tests listed under Plan C, they are nondiagnostic in nature. Because of the sophistication of the tests listed in Plans A and B, Table 3.2, they cannot be used for home testing. Some of the tests in Plan C can be used at home but are not considered as accurate in their ability to assess cardiorespiratory fitness.

We realize that for everyone to go to their physician's office or other establishments (universities, YMCAs) to obtain a sophisticated exercise tolerance test is impractical for many persons. Even so, the diagnostic test should be mandatory for high-risk persons and strongly recommended for sedentary persons who are more than 35 years of age. Once the diagnosis is made and the participant begins his or her program, less sophisticated tests can often be used for future evaluations. If one has any difficulty deciding what to do, a physician should be consulted and, if available in the community, an expert in evaluation and fitness. Along with your physician, many of your local YMCAs, Jewish Community Centers, and local colleges and universities have experts in adult fitness who can give the participant good advice.

SPECIFIC TEST ITEMS. Appendix A describes in detail a variety of test protocols for Plans A, B, and C, Table 3.2. The tests include protocols that can be administered on a motor-driven treadmill, work bicycle, and bench step. Also in Appendix A are recommendations for emergency procedures, special considerations in the selection of tests and testing personnel, and some helpful hints on administering tests.

Table 3.3 shows estimated functional capacity expressed as maximum oxygen uptake or METS, for several of the maximal exercise test protocols, and the one-and-one-half-mile run field test. Caution should be taken when using this table to estimate functional capacity. First, there is some variation from person to person on these tests; and, second, the treadmill or run time may be spuriously low for persons unaccustomed to taking a test. Therefore, for best results, prior practice is recommended.

The main concern in the evaluation process is that the participant is tested safely and properly, and ends up with a good estimate of functional capacity (fitness category). With the participant placed into the correct fitness category (Table 3.3), an accurate exercise prescription can be developed (see Section 4 on exercise prescription).

If the participant is of low risk and less than 35 years of age, then the three-minute step test described in Appendix A, p. 252, is probably the most practical test to self-administer at home. Once maximal oxygen uptake is estimated from the step test results, (Table A.21, Appendix A), then turn to Table 3.3 for fitness category determination.

If the participant wants to take a submaximal bicycle test, he or she should go to their local YMCA, health club, or university. They usually will have the equipment and administrative personnel available for help and advice.

The field-type test was designed to estimate maximum oxygen uptake on large groups of healthy young men and women. The most widely used field tests are the 12-minute and 1.5-mile runs. Both have a moderate to high relationship to the laboratory determined maximum oxygen uptake. Because the two tests have a very high intercorrelation and because the one-and-one-half-mile run test is easier to administer, only the one-and-one-half-mile test will be discussed.

Like other unmonitored tests, the field test should not be used as a diagnostic tool and should only be administered to healthy, young persons. An exception to this would be its use with trained middle-aged participants who have already been thoroughly evaluated for heart disease and potential risk. Best results are found when participants have had a few weeks of preliminary training. This allows time for some adaptation to training and practice in pacing oneself. Table 3.3 shows the estimation of maximum oxygen uptake based on the time to run one-and-one-half miles.

TABLE 3.3 Fitness classifications for exercise prescription for various levels of cardiorespiratory endurance

FITNESS CLASSIFICATION	Maximum Oxygen Uptake	
	ML/KG·MIN	METS*
1	17.5	5.0
	21.0	6.0
	24.5	7.0
	27.0	7.7
2	29.0	8.3
	31.5	9.0
	35.0	10.0
3	37.0	10.6
	39.0	11.1
	41.0	11.7
4	42.5	12.1
	45.0	12.9
	46.5	13.1
5	48.0	13.7
	49.5	13.9
	51.5	14.4
6	53.0	15.1
	55.0	15.7
	56.5	16.1
	58.0	16.6
7	60.0	17.1
	63.5	18.1
	66.0	18.9
	68.0	19.4
8	71.5	20.4
	74.0	21.1
	77.5	22.1

*MET refers to metabolic equivalent above the resting metabolic level. Value at rest is approximately 3.5 milliliters per kilogram of body weight per minute oxygen consumed.

**Data expressed in minutes and seconds of test protocol (duration) completed.

Mode of Estimating Maximum Oxygen Uptake

BALKE**	BRUCE**	ÅSTRAND	1.5 MILE RUN**
4:00	3:30	(mph)	(min:sec)
6:00	4:30		
8:00	6:00		
9:30	7:00	5.00	19:00
10:00	7:30	5.00	18:30
12:00	8:00	5.25	16:30
14:30	9:00	5.50	15:00
16:00	9:30	5.50	13.30
17:00	10:00	5.75	13:00
18:00	10:30	6.00	12:30
19:00	11:00	6.25	12:00
21:00	11:30	6.50	11:00
22:00	12:00	6.75	10:45
23:00	12:30	7.00	10:30
24:00	13:00	7.00	10:00
25:00	13:30	7.25	9:45
26:30	14:00	7.50	9:30
27:15	14:30	7.75	9:15
28:00	15:00	8.00	9:00
28:30	15:30	8.25	8:30
29:00	16:00	8.50	8:15
30:00	17:00	9.00	7:45
31:00	17:30	9.25	7:15
32:00	18:00	9.50	7:00
33:00	18:30	10.00	6:45
34:00	19:00	10.50	6:30
36:00	21:00	11.00	6:10

BODY COMPOSITION. The individual's body composition can be most accurately estimated by the underwater weighing technique (see Figure 3.1). Also, the underwater weighing technique can be administered out of the laboratory in a swimming pool. The underwater weighing technique is based on the Archimedes' principle of determining body density. The principle states that "A solid heavier than a fluid, if placed in it, descends to the bottom of the fluid, and the solid will, when weighed in the fluid, be lighter than its true weight by the weight of the fluid displaced." In other words, an object placed in water must be buoyed up by a counterforce that equals the weight of the water it displaces. The density of bone and muscle tissue are higher than water (1.2 to 3.0), while fat is less dense than water (0.90). Therefore, a person with more bone and muscle mass will weigh heavier in water and thus have a higher body density (lower percent fat).

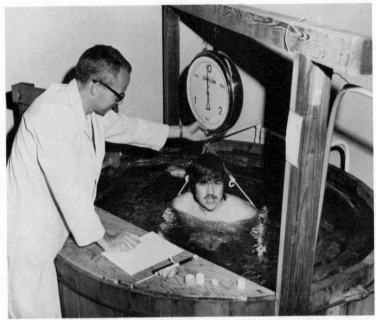

FIGURE 3.1. Underwater weighing technique conducted in a water tank.

Although quite accurate, determining body fat by the underwater weighing technique is not very practical. Therefore, anthropometric measurements (skinfold fat, girth, and diameter measures) are used to estimate the various components of body composition, that is, body density, relative or absolute fat, and lean body weight (bone and muscle). Skinfold thicknesses, body diameters or breadths, and body circumferences or girths have been used in the past with reasonable accuracy to estimate body composition. This technique correlates well with the underwater weighing method and has several advantages. The equipment is inexpensive, needs little or no space, and the measures can be easily and quickly obtained. Therefore, it can be used rather efficiently in testing large groups of people.

The anatomical landmarks for the various skinfold fat and girth sites are illustrated in Figures 3.2 and 3.3. A special caliper is used

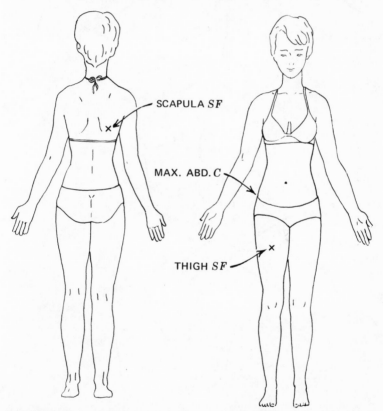

FIGURE 3.2. Skinfold measurement sites. (Courtesy of Behnke and Wilmore, 1974.)

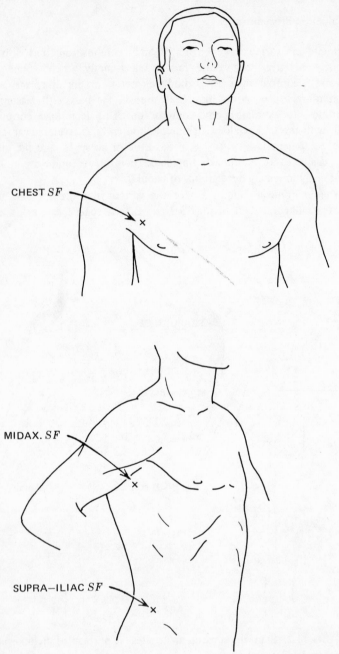

FIGURE 3.3. Skinfold measurement sites. (Courtesy of Behnke and Wilmore, 1974.)

to assess the fat that lies directly beneath the skin.* The skinfold is grasped firmly by the thumb and index finger, and the caliper is placed on the exact site approximately 1/4 to 1/2 inch from the thumb and finger (see Figure 3.4).

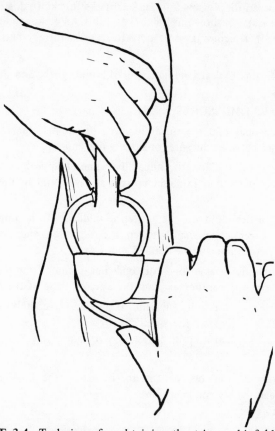

FIGURE 3.4. Technique for obtaining the triceps skinfold thickness. (Courtesy of Behnke and Wilmore, 1974.)

* The Harpenden caliper, Quinton Instruments, #3496, 2121 Terry Ave., Seattle, WA 98121; or Lange caliper, Cambridge Scientific Industries, 101 Virginia Ave., Cambridge, MD 21613.

A flexible steel tape is generally used for taking girth measures. The tape should be approximately two yards in length (two meters), have both English and metric units, and be easily retractable. A sliding broad-breadth caliper (anthropometer) is used for assessing diameters. A detailed description of anatomical landmarks for skinfold, girth, and diameter measures is shown in Table 3.4. Table A.24, Appendix A has an example of a recording sheet used to record anthropometric measures.

TABLE 3.4. Anatomical landmarks for skinfold, girth, and diameter measures

SKINFOLD FAT MEASURES:

Chest, diagonal fold one-third (women) or one-half (men) of the distance between the anterior-axillary line and nipple.

Axilla, vertical fold on the midaxillary line at approximately the level of the nipple (xiphoid process at lower end of the breast bone).

Triceps, vertical fold on the posterior midline of the upper arm (over triceps), halfway between the acromion and olecranon process with the elbow extended and relaxed.

Subscapular, fold taken on a diagonal line coming from the vertebral border 1 centimeter from the inferior angle of the scapula.

Abdominal, vertical fold adjacent to and approximately 2 centimeters laterally from the umbilicus.

Suprailiac, diagonal fold on the crest of the ilium at the midaxillary line.

Thigh, vertical fold on the anterior aspect of the thigh midway between the hip and knee joints.

GIRTH MEASURES:

Shoulder, taken in the horizontal plane at the maximum circumference of the shoulders at the level of the greatest lateral protrusion of the deltoid muscles.

Chest—high, taken in the horizontal plane at the largest circumference above the breasts (women).

Chest-Middle, taken in the horizontal plane at the maximum circumference.

Chest-low, taken in the horizontal plane just below the breast (women).

Abdominal, taken in a horizontal plane at the smallest circumference in the abdominal region, generally two to four inches above the umbilicus.

Waist, taken in the horizontal plane at the level of the umbilicus.

Gluteal, taken in the horizontal plane at the largest circumference around the buttocks. Subjects stand with feet together and gluteals tensed.

Thigh, taken in the horizontal plane just below the gluteal fold or maximal thigh girth.

Calf, taken in the horizontal plane at the maximum girth of the calf with muscle tensed.

Ankle, taken in the horizontal plane at the smallest point above the malleoli.

Arm, taken at maximal girth of the midarm when flexed to the greatest angle with the underlying muscles fully contracted.

Forearm, taken at the largest circumference with the forearm parallel to the floor, the elbow joint at a 90-degree angle, the hand in the supinated position, and the muscle flexed.

Wrist, taken over the styloid process of the radius and ulna with the arm extended in front of the body and fist clenched, relaxed, and pronated.

DIAMETER MEASURES:

Shoulder, distance between the outermost protrusions of the shoulder (deltoid muscles).

Biacromial, distance between the most lateral projections of the acromial processes.

Chest, arms abducted slightly for placement of the anthropometer at the level of the xiphoid process.

Bi-iliac, distance between the most lateral projections of the iliac crests.

Bitrochanter, distance between the most lateral projections of the greater trochanters.

Knee, 45-degree angle measurement at the smallest width of the knee, which is taken with the right foot placed on a small stool so that the knee is at a 90-degree angle.

Wrist, distance between the radial and ulna styloid processes.

Tables 3.5 to 3.8 list a series of equations using only skinfold fat measurements for different ages and sexes. Select the equation that best represents the population to be tested (male or female, young or middle-aged). The reason for so many different equations is because age and degree of fatness affect the results of the equations. Thus, equations for predicting body fat are population specific.

To calculate body fat from these conversion tables, match the measured variables with the conversion factors, and then place the conversions in the space marked conversions for each respective variable. Add or subtract these values to get body density. To convert density to percent fat, refer to Table 3.9. For example, if a young woman had skinfold fat of 24 and 20 millimeters, respectively, for the suprailiac and thigh, that would represent 1.0660 and 0.0220 conversion factors as listed in Table 3.6. Then subtract 0.0220 from 1.0660. Body density would be 1.0440, which converts to 24.14 percent fat (Table 3.9).

A simpler technique for determining relative body fat exists for men. Take the waist girth, holding the tape measure horizontal at the level of the umbilicus. Using Figures 3.5, determine relative fat from the body weight and waist girth. The example provided illustrates that a 170 pound man with a 34 inch waist would be 18 percent fat. Unfortunately, a similar simplified equation does not exist for women.

As mentioned earlier, there are many equations available that predict body fat from anthropometric measures. These equations were also shown to be population specific, as to age, sex, and degree of fatness. A third, and important, factor is that the best predictions of body fat have come from equations that included a variety of skinfold fat, girth, and diameter measures. The equations shown in Tables 3.5 to 3.8 and Figure 3.5 were selected for their simplicity as well as accuracy. If more time and other equipment, for example, a steel tape and anthropometer are available, slightly more accurate equations can be found in Appendix A, Tables A.25 to A.28. An equation that was found to be accurate with very lean men (distance runners) is also found in Appendix A, Table A.29.

TABLE 3.5. Conversion table for prediction of percent of body fat for young men[a,b]

CHEST SKINFOLD (mm)	CONVERSION FACTOR	SUBSCAPULAR SKINFOLD (mm)	CONVERSION FACTOR	THIGH SKINFOLD (mm)	CONVERSION FACTOR
1	1.90651	1	0.00055	1	0.0008
2	1.09586	2	0.00110	2	0.0016
3	1.09521	3	0.00165	3	0.0024
4	1.09456	4	0.00220	4	0.0032
5	1.09391	5	0.00275	5	0.0040
6	1.09326	6	0.00330	6	0.0048
7	1.09261	7	0.00385	7	0.0056
8	1.09196	8	0.00440	8	0.0064
9	1.09131	9	0.00495	9	0.0072
10	1.09066	10	0.00550	10	0.0080
11	1.09001	11	0.00605	11	0.0088
12	1.08936	12	0.00660	12	0.0096
13	1.08871	13	0.00715	13	0.0104
14	1.08806	14	0.00770	14	0.0112
15	1.08741	15	0.00825	15	0.0120
16	1.08676	16	0.00880	16	0.0128
17	1.08611	17	0.00935	17	0.0136
18	1.08546	18	0.00990	18	0.0144
19	1.08481	19	0.01045	19	0.0152
20	1.08416	20	0.01100	20	0.0160
21	1.08351	21	0.01155	21	0.0168
22	1.08286	22	0.01210	22	0.0176
23	1.08221	23	0.01265	23	0.0184
24	1.08156	24	0.01320	24	0.0192
25	1.08091	25	0.01375	25	0.0200
26	1.08026	26	0.01430	26	0.0208
27	1.07961	27	0.01485	27	0.0216
28	1.07896	28	0.01540	28	0.0224
29	1.07831	29	0.01595	29	0.0232
30	1.07766	30	0.01650	30	0.0240
31	1.07701	31	0.01705	31	0.0248
32	1.07636	32	0.01760	32	0.0256
33	1.07571	33	0.01815	33	0.0265
34	1.07506	34	0.01870	34	0.0272
35	1.07441	35	0.01925	35	0.0280
36	1.07376	36	0.01980	36	0.0288
37	1.07311	37	0.02035	37	0.0296
38	1.07246	38	0.02090	38	0.0304
39	1.07181	39	0.02145	39	0.0312
40	1.07116	40	0.02200	40	0.0320
41	1.07051	41	0.02255	41	0.0328
42	1.06986	42	0.02310	42	0.0336
43	1.06921	43	0.02365	43	0.0344
44	1.06856	44	0.02420	44	0.0352
45	1.06791	45	0.02475	45	0.0360
46	1.06726	46	0.02530	46	0.0368
47	1.06661	47	0.02585	47	0.0376
48	1.06596	48	0.02640	48	0.0384
49	1.06531	49	0.02695	49	0.0392
50	1.06466	50	0.02750	50	0.0400

[a]Table developed by M.L. Pollock (Institute for Aerobics Research) and A.J. Jackson (University of Houston).
[b]Pollock, Hickman, Kendrick, Jackson, Linnerud, and Dawson. "Prediction of body density in young and middle-aged men." *J. Appl. Physiol.*, 40:300-304 (1976).

Density = 1.09716 - 0.00065 × chest - 0.00055 × subscapular - 0.0008 × thigh
R = 0.82 Standard error = 0.0080

See the following page for individual conversion.

TABLE 3.5. (Continued) Personal measurement and conversion form for determining body fat for young men [a]

YOUNG MEN

PERSONAL MEASUREMENTS

Chest _____ mm

Subscapular_____mm

Thigh _____ mm

CONVERSIONS

Chest _____

  −

Subscapular_____

  −

Thigh _____

  =

Density _____
  (gm/cc)

(Density is the sum of
conversion factors.)

[a]Use this form to record personal measurements for calculation of body density. Conversion factors are from previous page. To convert density to percent fat refer to Table 3.9.

TABLE 3.6. Conversion table for prediction of percent body fat for young women[a,b]

SUPRAILIAC SKINFOLD (mm)	CONVERSION FACTOR	THIGH SKINFOLD (mm)	CONVERSION FACTOR
1	1.0844	1	0.0011
2	1.0836	2	0.0022
3	1.0828	3	0.0033
4	1.0820	4	0.0044
5	1.0812	5	0.0055
6	1.0804	6	0.0066
7	1.0796	7	0.0077
8	1.0788	8	0.0088
9	1.0780	9	0.0099
10	1.0772	10	0.0110
11	1.0764	11	0.0121
12	1.0756	12	0.0132
13	1.0748	13	0.0143
14	1.0740	14	0.0154
15	1.0732	15	0.0165
16	1.0724	16	0.0176
17	1.0716	17	0.0187
18	1.0708	18	0.0198
19	1.0700	19	0.0209
20	1.0692	20	0.0220
21	1.0684	21	0.0231
22	1.0676	22	0.0242
23	1.0668	23	0.0253
24	1.0660	24	0.0264
25	1.0652	25	0.0275
26	1.0644	26	0.0286
27	1.0636	27	0.0297
28	1.0628	28	0.0308
29	1.0620	29	0.0319
30	1.0612	30	0.0330
31	1.0604	31	0.0341
32	1.0596	32	0.0352
33	1.0588	33	0.0363
34	1.0580	34	0.0374
35	1.0572	35	0.0385
36	1.0564	36	0.0396
37	1.0556	37	0.0407
38	1.0548	38	0.0418
39	1.0540	39	0.0429
40	1.0532	40	0.0440
41	1.0524	41	0.0451
42	1.0516	42	0.0462
43	1.0508	43	0.0473
44	1.0500	44	0.0484
45	1.0492	45	0.0495
46	1.0484	46	0.0506
47	1.0476	47	0.0517
48	1.0468	48	0.0528
49	1.0460	49	0.0539
50	1.0452	50	0.0550

[a]Table developed by M.L. Pollock (Institute for Aerobics Research) and A.J. Jackson (University of Houston).

[b]Pollock, Laughridge, Coleman, Linnerud, and Jackson. "Prediction of body density in young and middle-aged women." *J. Appl. Physiol. 38*: 745-749 (1975).
Density = 1.0852 - 0.0008 × suprailiac - 0.0011 × thigh
R = 0.775 Standard error = 0.0091

See the following page for individual conversion.

TABLE 3.6. (Continued) Personal measurement and conversion form for determining body fat for young women [a]

YOUNG WOMEN

PERSONAL MEASUREMENTS

Suprailiac _____ mm

Thigh _____ mm

CONVERSIONS

Suprailiac _____

−

Thigh _____

=

Density _____
  (gm/cc)

(Density is the sum of
conversion factors.)

[a]Use this form to record personal measurements for calculation of body density. Conversion factors are from previous page. To convert density to percent fat refer to Table 3.9.

TABLE 3.7. Conversion table for prediction of percent body fat for middle-aged men[a,b]

CHEST SKINFOLD (mm)	CONVERSION FACTOR	AXILLA SKINFOLD (mm)	CONVERSION FACTOR
1	1.07562	1	0.00053
2	1.07464	2	0.00106
3	1.07366	3	0.00159
4	1.07268	4	0.00212
5	1.07170	5	0.00265
6	1.07072	6	0.00318
7	1.06974	7	0.00371
8	1.06876	8	0.00424
9	1.06778	9	0.00477
10	1.06680	10	0.00530
11	1.06582	11	0.00583
12	1.06484	12	0.00636
13	1.06386	13	0.00689
14	1.06288	14	0.00742
15	1.06190	15	0.00795
16	1.06092	16	0.00848
17	1.05994	17	0.00901
18	1.05896	18	0.00954
19	1.05798	19	0.01007
20	1.05700	20	0.01060
21	1.05602	21	0.01113
22	1.05504	22	0.01166
23	1.05406	23	0.01219
24	1.05308	24	0.01272
25	1.05210	25	0.01325
26	1.05112	26	0.01378
27	1.05014	27	0.01431
28	1.04916	28	0.01484
29	1.04818	29	0.01537
30	1.04720	30	0.01590
31	1.04622	31	0.01643
32	1.04524	32	0.01696
33	1.04426	33	0.01749
34	1.04328	34	0.01802
35	1.04230	35	0.01855
36	1.04132	36	0.01908
37	1.04034	37	0.01961
38	1.03936	38	0.02014
39	1.03838	39	0.02067
40	1.03740	40	0.02120
41	1.03642	41	0.02173
42	1.03544	42	0.02226
43	1.03446	43	0.02279
44	1.03348	44	0.02332
45	1.03250	45	0.02385
46	1.03152	46	0.02438
47	1.03054	47	0.02491
48	1.02956	48	0.02544
49	1.02858	49	0.02597
50	1.02760	50	0.02650

[a]Table developed by M.L. Pollock (Institute for Aerobics Research) and A.J. Jackson (University of Houston).
[b]Pollock, Hickman, Kendrick, Jackson, Linnerud, and Dawson. "Prediction of body density in young and middle-aged men." *J. Appl. Physiol.*, 40:300-304 (1976).

Density = 1.0766 - 0.00098 × chest - 0.00053 × axilla
R = 0.78 Standard error = 0.0082

See the following page for individual conversion.

TABLE 3.7. (Continued) Personal measurement and conversion form for determining body fat for middle-aged men[a]

MIDDLE-AGED MEN

PERSONAL MEASUREMENTS

Chest _____ mm

Axilla _____ mm

CONVERSIONS

Chest _____

—

Axilla _____

=

Density _____
(gm/cc)

(Density is the sum of
conversion factors.)

[a]Use this form to record personal measurements for calculation of body density. Conversion factors are from previous page. To convert density to percent fat refer to Table 3.9.

TABLE 3.8. Conversion table for prediction of percent body fat for middle-aged women[a,b]

AXILLA SKINFOLD (mm)	CONVERSION FACTOR	THIGH SKINFOLD (mm)	CONVERSION FACTOR
1	1.0742	1	0.0007
2	1.0730	2	0.0014
3	1.0718	3	0.0021
4	1.0706	4	0.0028
5	1.0694	5	0.0035
6	1.0682	6	0.0042
7	1.0670	7	0.0049
8	1.0658	8	0.0056
9	1.0646	9	0.0063
10	1.0634	10	0.0070
11	1.0622	11	0.0077
12	1.0610	12	0.0084
13	1.0598	13	0.0091
14	1.0586	14	0.0098
15	1.0574	15	0.0105
16	1.0562	16	0.0112
17	1.0550	17	0.0119
18	1.0538	18	0.0126
19	1.0526	19	0.0133
20	1.0514	20	0.0140
21	1.0502	21	0.0147
22	1.0490	22	0.0154
23	1.0478	23	0.0161
24	1.0466	24	0.0168
25	1.0454	25	0.0175
26	1.0442	26	0.0182
27	1.0430	27	0.0189
28	1.0418	28	0.0196
29	1.0406	29	0.0203
30	1.0394	30	0.0210
31	1.0382	31	0.0217
32	1.0370	32	0.0224
33	1.0358	33	0.0231
34	1.0346	34	0.0238
35	1.0334	35	0.0245
36	1.0322	36	0.0252
37	1.0310	37	0.0259
38	1.0298	38	0.0266
39	1.0286	39	0.0273
40	1.0274	40	0.0280
41	1.0262	41	0.0287
42	1.0250	42	0.0294
43	1.0238	43	0.0301
44	1.0226	44	0.0308
45	1.0214	45	0.0315
46	1.0202	46	0.0322
47	1.0190	47	0.0329
48	1.0178	48	0.0336
49	1.0166	49	0.0343
50	1.0154	50	0.0350

[a]Table developed by M.L. Pollock (Institute for Aerobics Research) and A.J. Jackson (University of Houston).

[b]Pollock, Laughridge, Coleman, Linnerud, and Jackson. "Prediction of body density in young and middle-aged women." *J. Appl. Physiol., 38*:745-749 (1975).

Density = $1.0754 - 0.0012 \times$ axilla $- 0.0007 \times$ thigh

$R = 0.856$ Standard error = 0.0076

See the following page for individual conversion.

TABLE 3.8. (Continued) Personal measurement and conversion form for determining body fat for middle-aged women[a]

MIDDLE-AGED WOMEN

PERSONAL MEASUREMENTS

Axilla _____ mm

Thigh _____ mm

CONVERSIONS

Axilla _____

—

Thigh _____

=

Density _____
(gm/cc)

(Density is the sum of
conversion factors.)

[a]Use this form to record personal measurements for calculation of body density. Conversion factors are from previous page. To convert density to percent fat refer to Table 3.9.

TABLE 3.9. Table to convert density to percent fat[a]

Name: _____ Date: _____ / _____ / _____

DENSITY	PERCENT FAT	DENSITY	PERCENT FAT	DENSITY	PERCENT FAT
1.000	45.00	1.033	29.19	1.066	14.35
1.001	44.51	1.034	28.72	1.067	13.92
1.002	44.01	1.035	28.26	1.068	13.48
1.003	43.52	1.036	27.80	1.069	13.05
1.004	43.03	1.037	27.34	1.070	12.62
1.005	42.54	1.038	26.88	1.071	12.18
1.006	42.05	1.039	26.42	1.072	11.75
1.007	41.56	1.040	25.96	1.073	11.32
1.008	41.07	1.041	25.50	1.074	10.89
1.009	40.58	1.042	25.05	1.075	10.47
1.010	40.10	1.043	24.59	1.076	10.04
1.011	39.61	1.044	24.14	1.077	9.61
1.012	39.13	1.045	23.68	1.078	9.18
1.013	38.65	1.046	23.23	1.079	8.76
1.014	38.17	1.047	22.78	1.080	8.33
1.015	37.68	1.048	22.33	1.081	7.91
1.016	37.20	1.049	21.88	1.082	7.49
1.017	36.73	1.050	21.43	1.083	7.06
1.018	36.25	1.051	20.98	1.084	6.64
1.019	35.77	1.052	20.53	1.085	6.22
1.020	35.29	1.053	20.09	1.086	5.80
1.021	34.82	1.054	19.64	1.087	5.38
1.022	34.34	1.055	19.19	1.088	4.96
1.023	33.87	1.056	18.75	1.089	4.55
1.024	33.40	1.057	18.31	1.090	4.13
1.025	32.93	1.058	17.86	1.091	3.71
1.026	32.46	1.059	17.42	1.092	3.30
1.027	31.99	1.060	16.98	1.093	2.88
1.028	31.52	1.061	16.54	1.094	2.47
1.029	31.05	1.062	16.10	1.095	2.05
1.030	30.58	1.063	15.66	1.096	1.64
1.031	30.12	1.064	15.23	1.097	1.23
1.032	29.65	1.065	14.79	1.098	0.82

DENSITY _____ PERCENT FAT _____
(Sum of conversions)

[a]Siri Percent Fat Formula: % Fat = $\dfrac{4.950}{\text{density}} - 4.50 \times 100$

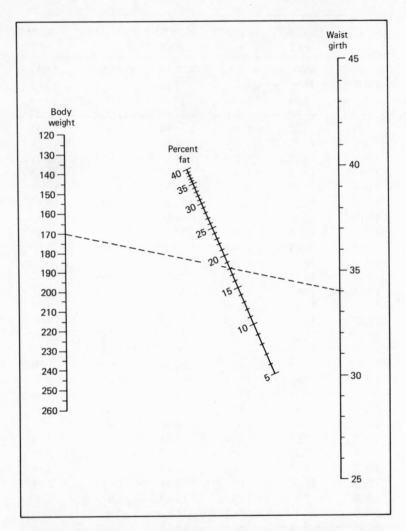

FIGURE 3.5. Prediction of relative body fat in men from waist girth and body weight. (Courtesy of Dr. Brian J. Sharkey, University of Montana, Missoula, MO)

STRENGTH. Strength can be easily assessed by the one-repetition maximum test (1-RM). The basic muscle or muscle group to be tested is selected and then individuals are given a series of trials to determine the greatest weight they can lift just once for that particular lift. This test is conducted largely through trial and error when they are inexperienced in lifting weights. Start with a weight that individuals can lift comfortably, then keep adding weight until they can lift the weight correctly just one time. If they can lift this weight more than once, more weight needs to be added until a true 1-RM is reached. Although 1-RMs can be obtained for any basic weight training exercise, test batteries usually select three or four exercises that represent the body's major muscle groups. Table 3.10 gives a series of values for selected strength exercises for both males and females on the basis of body weight. While the strength requirements will differ by each sport or activity, or even by position or event within each sport, these values represent optimal values for the average person who is training mainly for general fitness purposes. Specific standards for each sport have yet to be developed.

Additional strength tests are available using dynamometers, cable tensiometers, and elaborate force transducers and recorders. These tests, however, require expensive equipment and do not always provide a substantial improvement in measurement accuracy. Reference to a recent text in measurement and evaluation, for example, Baumgartner and Jackson, will provide additional information on these laboratory types of tests.

MUSCULAR ENDURANCE. Muscular endurance has been measured in a number of different ways, including the greatest number of sit-ups that can be performed in a fixed period of time (usually 30 seconds or 1 minute), or the maximum number of pushups, pull-ups, or bar dips that can be performed continuously in an indefinite time period. Many of these tests penalize the participant who has long legs, short arms, or a heavy body weight. To eliminate this, a concept has evolved that uses a fixed percentage of the individual's body weight as the resistance, and the individual lifts this as many times as possible until he or she reaches the point of fatigue or exhaustion. Firm guidelines have yet to be established with regard to what the actual fixed percentages of the individual's body weight should be for each of the muscle groups tested. In fact, it is debatable whether the weight used in the

TABLE 3.10. Optimal strength values for various body weights (based on the 1-RM test)[a,b]

BODY WEIGHT (lb)	BENCH PRESS MALE	BENCH PRESS FEMALE	STANDING PRESS MALE	STANDING PRESS FEMALE	CURL MALE	CURL FEMALE	LEG PRESS MALE	LEG PRESS FEMALE
80	80	56	53	37	40	28	160	112
100	100	70	67	47	50	35	200	140
120	120	84	80	56	60	42	240	168
140	140	98	93	65	70	49	280	196
160	160	112	107	75	80	56	320	224
180	180	126	120	84	90	63	360	252
200	200	140	133	93	100	70	400	280
220	220	154	147	103	110	77	440	308
240	240	168	160	112	120	84	480	336

[a]Note—Data collected on Universal Gym apparatus. Information collected on other apparatus could modify results.
[b]Data express in pounds.

test should be a fixed percentage of the individual's body weight or a fixed percentage of the individual's 1-RM or absolute strength. As an example, if the endurance test for the bench press movement was conducted using 50 percent of the individual's body weight as the resistance, the 180-pound man would be asked to lift 90 pounds as many times as he could. A strong man of this body weight would be able to lift this 90-pound weight 20 or more times, while the relatively weak man who weighs 180 pounds may not be able to lift the 90-pound weight even one single repetition, that is, the designated weight exceeds his 1-RM. In this case, the test for muscular endurance would be highly dependent on strength. To isolate muscular endurance as a pure component, where the test is not so dependent on the individual's strength, it is advocated that the test battery be established on the basis of the individual's strength, and not body weight.

In accordance with the above recommendation, it is suggested that a fixed percentage of 70 percent of the maximum strength be used to test muscle endurance. This percentage would be the same for all movements tested. Since this is a relatively new concept, norms or standards have yet to be established but could be easily developed for each specific population to be tested. On the basis of limited test data, the recreational athlete or health seeking exerciser should be able to perform 12 to 15 repetitions and the competitive athlete, 20 to 25 repetitions at 70 percent of his or her maximum strength for each of the movements tested.

Two tests that have been traditionally used to measure muscular endurance are the pushup and sit-up tests, to assess upper body and abdominal muscular endurance, respectively. The pushup test is administered with the individual in the standard "up" position for a full pushup (Figure 3.6). The tester places his or her fist on the floor beneath the individual's chest, and the individual must lower himself down until his chest touches the tester's fist, keeping his back straight, and then raising back to the up position. The maximum number of correctly performed pushups is counted and then compared to Table 3.11, which lists standards relative to age and sex. Women can perform this test from the bent-knee position (Figure 3.7).

In the sit-up test, the individual starts by lying on his back, knees bent, heels flat on the floor, and hands interlocked behind the neck. The tester holds the individual's feet down. The individual performs as many correct sit-ups (Figure 3.8a) as possible in a 60-second period.

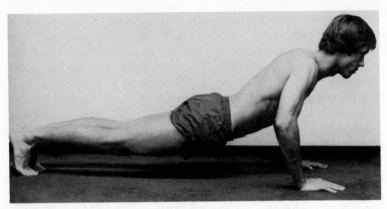

FIGURE 3.6. Standard or full pushup.

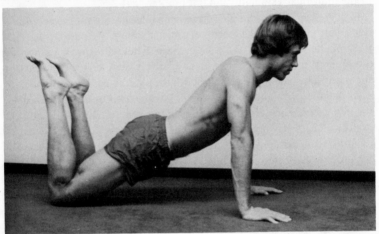

FIGURE 3.7. Modified pushup.

Elbows should be touched to the knees in the up position, and this must be followed by a complete return to the full lying position prior to starting the next sit-up (Figure 3.8b). The total number of sit-ups performed in 60 seconds is recorded and compared to Table 3.12, which lists standards relative to age and sex.

TABLE 3.11. Pushup muscular endurance test standards[a]

| AGE | MALES | | | | | | FEMALES[b] | | | | | |
	EXCELLENT	GOOD	AVERAGE	FAIR	POOR	EXCELLENT	GOOD	AVERAGE	FAIR	POOR
20-29	55-above	45-54	35-44	20-34	0-19	49-above	34-48	17-33	6-16	0-5
30-39	45-above	35-44	25-34	15-24	0-14	40-above	25-39	12-24	4-11	0-3
40-49	40-above	30-39	20-29	12-19	0-11	35-above	20-34	8-19	3-7	0-2
50-59	35-above	25-34	15-24	8-14	0-7	30-above	15-29	6-14	2-5	0-1
60-69	30-above	20-29	10-19	5-9	0-4	20-above	5-19	3-4	1-2	0

[a]These values represent approximations, since actual norms are not available.
[b]Modified pushup.

TABLE 3.12. Sit-up muscular endurance test standards[a,b]

AGE	MALES					FEMALES				
	EXCELLENT	GOOD	AVERAGE	FAIR	POOR	EXCELLENT	GOOD	AVERAGE	FAIR	POOR
20-29	48-above	43-47	37-42	33-36	0-32	44-above	39-43	33-38	29-32	0-28
30-39	40-above	35-39	29-34	25-28	0-24	36-above	31-35	25-30	21-24	0-20
40-49	35-above	30-34	24-29	20-23	0-19	31-above	26-30	19-25	16-18	0-15
50-59	30-above	25-29	19-24	15-18	0-14	26-above	21-25	15-20	11-14	0-10
60-69	25-above	20-24	14-19	10-13	0-9	21-above	16-20	10-15	6-9	0-5

[a]These values represent approximations, since actual norms are not available.

[b]Test is timed for 60-seconds.

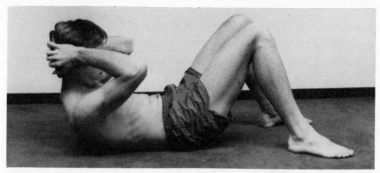

FIGURE 3.8a. Starting and ending position for the 60-second, sit-up test.

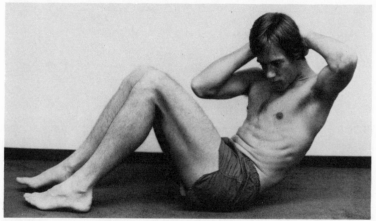

FIGURE 3.8b. The sit and reach test to determine flexibility at the hip joint.

FLEXIBILITY. Probably the most accurate tests of flexibility presently available are those that assess the actual range of motion of the various joints. Although this is easily accomplished by instruments such as the Leighton Flexometer and the electrogoniometer, these pieces of equipment are not readily available.

Since flexibility is specific to each joint, no generalized flexibility test is available. Because the emphasis of this book is on adult physical fitness and related health aspects, lower back flexibility will be mentioned here. As stated earlier, low back pain and disability are prevalent among men and women in the adult population. Much of this problem is related to the lack of flexibility in the back of the legs (hamstrings), hips, and lower back. To measure this area, a simple field test called the sit and reach test can be used (Figure 3.9).

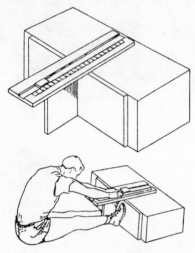

FIGURE 3.9. The sit and reach test to determine flexibility at the hip joint.

In the sit and reach test, the individual sits with the legs extended directly in front of him or her and the knees pressed against the floor. The feet are placed against a stool to which is attached a yardstick, with the 14-inch mark being placed at the point where the foot contacts the stool. The individual places the index fingers of both hands together and reaches forward slowly as far as possible. The distance reached is noted on the yardstick and recorded. The knees must be kept in contact with the floor and bouncing is to be discouraged. Standards for the normal population are presented in Table 3.13. Obviously, this test will be influenced by the length of the arms and legs of the individual, in addition to his or her flexibility.

SUMMARY

In this section we attempt to explain and discuss many of the factors involved in a comprehensive medical screening and physical fitness examination. In the first portion we talk about risk factors related to coronary heart disease and illustrate a coronary risk factor profile chart. Within this profile chart certain estimations are made as to high and low risk.

TABLE 3.13. Standards for the sit and reach flexibility test.

	SIT AND REACH
Excellent	22 in. or greater
Good	19-21 in.
Average	14-18 in.
Fair	12-13 in.
Poor	11 in. or less

From *Health Improvement Program,* National Athletic Health Institute, Inglewood, CA.

Later we describe tests to evaluate cardiorespiratory fitness, body composition (leanness-fatness), strength, muscular endurance, and flexibility. The recommended tests are graded as to their sophistication and feasibility. Easily administered tests are described in this section, while more extensive and sophisticated testing procedures are detailed in Appendix A.

An important aspect of this section is its ability to explain to the participants how to properly and safely assess their health and physical fitness status. This information should give participants a better basis for intiating an exercise program at the proper level or for monitoring the progress of the exercise program. In order to assess the status of physical fitness, norm tables that are specific to age and sex are shown. The age-specific norm tables are categorized for ages 20 to 29; 30 to 39; 40 to 49; 50 to 59; and 60-plus years.

REFERENCES

1. American College of Sports Medicine *Guidelines for Graded Exercise Testing and Exercise Prescription.* Philadelphia: Lea and Febiger, 1975.

2. American Heart Association. *Exercise Testing and Training of Apparently Healthy Individuals: A Handbook for Physicians.* New York: American Heart Association, 1972.

3. American Heart Association. *Exercise Testing and Training of Individuals with Heart Disease or at High Risk for its Development: A Handbook for Physicians.* New York: American Heart Association, 1975.

4. Åstrand, P., I.A. Ryhming. "Nomogram for calculation of aerobic capacity from pulse rate during submaximal work." *J. Appl.*

Physiol., 7:218-221 (1954).

5. Åstrand, P.O., and K. Rodahl. *Textbook of Work Physiology*, 2nd Ed., New York:McGraw-Hill, 1977.

6. Balke, B., and R. Ware. "An experimental study of physical fitness of air force personnel." *U.S. Armed Forces Med. J., 10*:675-688 (1959).

7. Balke, B. "A simple field test for the assessment of physical fitness." *CARI Report 63-6*. Civil Aeromedical Research Institute, Federal Aviation Agency, Oklahoma City, 1963.

8. Baumgartner, T.A., and A. Jackson. *Measurement for Evaluation in Physical Education*. Boston: Houghton Mifflin, 1975.

9. Behnke, A.R., and J.H. Wilmore. *Evaluation and Regulation of Body Build and Composition*. Englewood Cliffs, N.J.: Prentice-Hall, 1974.

10. Blackburn, H. (ed.). *Measurement in Exercise Electrocardiography*. Springfield, Ill: C.C. Thomas Publisher, 1969.

11. Bruce, R.A., F. Kusumi, and D. Hosmer. "Maximal oxygen intake and nomographic assessment of functional aerobic impairment in cardiovascular disease." *Am. Heart J., 85*:546-562 (1973).

12. Cooper, K.H. "Correlation between field and treadmill testing as a means of assessing maximal oxygen intake." *JAMA, 203*:201-204 (1968).

13. Cooper, K.H. "Guidelines in the management of the exercising patient." *JAMA, 211*:1663-1667 (1970).

14. Cooper, K.H., J.G. Purdy, S.R. White, M.L. Pollock, and A.C. Linnerud. "Age-fitness adjusted maximal heart rates." In: *Medicine Sport*, Vol. 10, D. Brunner and E. Jokl (eds.). Basel, Switzerland: Karger, 1977, pp. 78-88.

15. Davis, J.A., and V.A. Convertino. "A comparison of heart rate methods for predicting endurance training intensity." *Med. Sci. Sports, 7*:295-298 (1975).

16. Disch, J., R. Frankiewicz, and A. Jackson. "Construct validation of distance run tests." *Res. Q., 46*:169-176 (1975).

17. Ellestad, M.H. *Stress Testing Principles and Practice*. Philadelphia: F.A. Davis Company, 1975.

18. Froelicher, V.F., H. Brammell, G. Davis, I. Noguera, A. Stewart, and M.C. Lancaster. "A comparison of the reproducibility and physiologic response to three maximal treadmill exercise protocols." *Chest, 65*:512-517 (1974).

19. Katch, F.I., and W.D. McArdle. *Nutrition, Weight Control, and Exercise.* Boston: Houghton Mifflin, 1977.

20. Kattus, A.A. "Physical training and beta-adrenergic blocking drugs in modifying coronary insufficiency." In: *Coronary Circulation and Energetics of the Myocardium,* G. Marchetti, and B. Toccardi (eds.). New York: Karger, 1967.

21. Karvonen, M., K. Kentala, and O. Muslala, "The effects of training heart rate: A longitudinal study." *Ann. Med. Exptl. Biol. Fenn., 35*:307-315 (1957).

22. McArdle, W.D., F.I. Katch, G.S. Pechar, L. Jacobson, and S. Ruck. "Reliability and interrelationships between maximal oxygen intake, physical work capacity, and step-test scores in college women." *Med. Sci. Sports, 4*:182-186 (1972).

23. Mitchell, J., B. Sproule, and C. Chapman. "The physiological meaning of the maximal oxygen intake test." *J. Clin. Invest., 37*:538-547 (1958).

24. Myers, C.R., L.A. Golding, and W.E. Sinning. (eds). *The Y's Way to Physical Fitness.* Emmaus, Pa.: Rodale Press, 1973.

25. Naughton, J., B. Balke, and F. Nagle. "Refinements in methods of evaluation and physical conditioning before and after myocardial infarction." *Amer. J. Cardiol., 14*:837 (1964).

26. Naughton, J.P., and H.K. Hellerstein, (eds). *Exercise Testing and exercise training in Coronary Heart Disease.* New York; Academic Press, 1973.

27. Pollock, M.L., H.S. Miller, A.C. Linnerud, C.L. Royster, W.E. Smith, and W.S. Sonner. "Physiological findings in well-trained middle-aged American men." *Brit. J. Sports Med., 7*:222-229 (1973).

28. Pollock, M.L., E.E. Laughridge, B. Coleman, A.C. Linnerud, and A. Jackson. "Prediction of body density in young and middle-aged women." *J. Appl. Physiol., 38*:745-749 (1975).

29. Pollock, M.L., R.L. Bohannon, K.H. Cooper, J.J. Ayres, A. Ward, S.R. White, and A.C. Linnerud, "A comparative analysis of four protocols for maximal treadmill stress testing." *Am. Heart J., 92*:39-46 (1976).

30. Pollock. M.L., T. Hickman, Z, Kendrick, A. Jackson, A.C. Linnerud, and G. Dawson. "Prediction of body density in young and middle-aged men." *J. Appl. Physiol., 40*:300-304 (1976).

31. Pollock, M.L., A. Jackson, J. Ayres, A. Ward., A.C. Linnerud, and L.R. Gettman. "Body composition of elite class distance runners." *Ann. NY Acad. Sci.* 307:361-370 (1977).

32. Rochmis, P., and H. Blackburn. "Exercise tests a survey of procedures, safety, and litigation experience in approximately 170,000 tests." *JAMA, 217*:1061-1066 (1971).

33. Taylor, H.E., E. Buskirk, and A. Henschel. "Maximal oxygen intake as an objective measure of cardiorespiratory performance." *J. Appl. Physiol., 8*:77-80 (1955).

34. Taylor, H.L., Y. Wang, L. Rowell, and G. Blomqvist. "The standardization and interpretation of submaximal and maximal tests of working capacity." *Pediatrics, 32*:(II):703-722 (1963).

35. Taylor, H.L., W. Haskell, S.M. Fox, III, and H. Blackburn. "Exercise tests: a summary of procedures and concepts of stress testing for cardiovascular diagnosis and function evaluation." In: *Measurement in Exercise Electrocardiography* H. Blackburn (ed.) Springfield: C.C. Thomas, 1969, pp 259-305.

36. Wilmore, J.H. *Athletic Training and Physical Fitness: Physiological Principles and Practices of the Conditioning Process.* Boston: Allyn and Bacon, 1977.

37. Wilson, P.K., (ed.). *Adult Fitness and Cardiac Rehabilitation.* Baltimore: University Park Press, 1975.

38. Wyndham, C.H. "Submaximal tests for estimating maximum oxygen intake." *Canad. Med. Ass. J., 96*:736-745 (1967).

Section 4
The Exercise Prescription

GUIDELINES AND PRELIMINARY CONSIDERATIONS

A clear understanding of the person involved is necessary in order to safely and adequately prescribe exercise. People vary greatly in status of health and fitness, structure, age, motivation, and needs; therefore, the individual approach to exercise prescription is recommended.

The needs and goals of elementary school children, college athletes, middle-aged men and women, and cardiac patients clearly differ. For example, an athlete often must get into condition quickly for a competition. In this case, many safeguards concerning intensity and progression of exercise are not closely followed. Although the abrupt approach is followed in certain instances, its general use is not recommended. The initial experience with endurance training should be of low to moderate intensity and progression that allows for gradual adaptation. On the basis of much experience with adult programs, the abrupt approach can result in discouraging future motivation for participation in endurance activities. Improper advice or prescription also can lead to undue muscle or joint strain or soreness, other orthopedic problems, undue fatigue, and risk of precipitating a heart attack. The latter is rare and occurs mainly with middle-aged and older participants. Most incidents have occurred because of the lack of appropriate previous medical evaluation and clearance, incorrect exercise prescription, inadequate supervision, or an extreme climatic condition such as excess heat and humidity or severe cold.

The following guidelines are suggested in the exercise prescription process.

Preliminary Suggestions

1. Have adequate medical information available to assess health status properly. This would include a medical history, physical examination, risk factor, and laboratory evaluations.

2. Have information concerning the present status of physical fitness and exercise habits.

3. Know the individual's needs, interests, and objectives for being in an exercise program.

4. Set realistic short-term and long-term goals.

5. Give advice on proper attire and equipment for an exercise program.

Suggestions for Initial Phases of an Exercise Program

1. Properly educate the participant in the principles of exercise, exercise prescription, and methods of monitoring and recording exercise experiences.

2. Give adequate physical leadership and direction in the early stages of the exercise program to assure proper implementation and progress.

3. Remember that *education*, *motivation*, and *leadership* are the keys to a successful exercise program.

Long-Term Suggestions

1. Reevaluations are necessary for reassessing individual status, functional physical fitness, and exercise prescription.

2. Reevaluations are also important in the education and motivation processes.

The program is prescribed as soon as the health and fitness status and needs and objectives of the participants are determined. Having this information, plus knowing the participants' activity interests and available time, the type and quantity of exercise may be determined. It is important for the initial exercise experience to be enjoyable, refreshing, and not too demanding either physiologically or time wise. The slow, gradual approach to initiating an exercise program will help culture a more positive attitude toward physical activity and enhance the probability of long-term adherence. Also, if the prescribed program is too demanding, adherence is not very likely. For more information on this subject, see Section 7.

CARDIORESPIRATORY ENDURANCE AND WEIGHT REDUCTION

The research findings reported in Section 2 described the amount of work considered necessary to develop and maintain an optimal level of cardiorespiratory endurance. Within certain limits, the total energy cost (calories utilized) of a training regimen is the most important factor in the development of cardiorespiratory endurance, and in weight reduction and control. For most people, this energy cost amounts to approximately 900 to 1500 calories per week or 300 to 500 calories per exercise session. Table 4.1 emphasizes the importance of frequency, intensity, and duration of training in attaining a certain level of calorie expenditure and gives general recommendations for exercise prescription.

TABLE 4.1. Recommendations for exercise prescription

1. Frequency	3 to 5 days per week
2. Intensity	60 to 90% of maximum heart rate
	50 to 80% of maximum oxygen uptake
3. Duration	15 to 60 minutes (continuous)
4. Mode-Activity	Run, jog, walk, bicycle, swim
	or endurance sport activities
5. Initial level of fitness	High = higher work load
	Low = lower work load

These recommendations are designed for the needs of the general population and not for highly trained endurance athletes or persons of low or poor health status, for example, cardiac patients or severely handicapped individuals. Competitive runners usually exercise daily and may cover in excess of 100 miles per week. On the other extreme, certain hazardous or debilitating diseases, such as coronary heart disease and arthritis, may greatly limit individuals in their training. See Section 5 for special considerations in cardiac rehabilitation.

FREQUENCY. Exercise should be performed on a regular basis from three to five days per week. Although programs of sufficient intensity and duration show some cardiorespiratory improvements with a frequency less than three days per week, little or no body weight or fat loss is found. Also, improvement in cardiorespiratory endurance is only minimal to modest in programs of less than three days per week (usually less than 10%). Participants in one- or two-day-per-week programs often complain that the workout sessions are too intermittent and break the continuity of the training regimen. Another common complaint is: "It seemed as though I was starting anew each time I came out." Our experience has shown that feelings such as these often lead to dropouts in a program. Under unusual conditions, if time and available facilities are important considerations, then one- or two-day-per-week regimens may be acceptable and serve a temporary purpose.

Conditioning every other day is most frequently recommended when initiating an endurance exercise regimen. Daily, vigorous exercise often becomes too demanding initially and does not allow enough time between workouts for the musculoskeletal system to adapt properly. This nonadaptive state generally leads to undesirable muscle soreness, fatigue, and possible injury. This guideline may seem to contradict the research findings reported in Section 2 and the recommendations for exercise prescription shown in Table 4.1. However, the data from young men running 30 minutes, five days per week, or 45 minutes, three days per week showed them to incur injuries at a significantly higher rate than they did on three-day-per-week programs of 15- and 30-minute durations. In fact, the men in the three-day-per-week programs had little or no injury problems. Most of the injuries that did occur concerned problems of the knee, shin, ankle, or foot.

Persons who are at a low level of fitness (cardiac patients, etc.) and whose initial programs are restricted to 5 to 15 minutes per session, may want to exercise twice each day and often every day. An example of this special condition is a person who is placed into a walking program of low intensity and short duration. In this case a person may adapt better to shorter, but more frequent exercise sessions. Another substitute for exercising every other day is to alternate the regular exercise session with days of very mild activity. For persons who are initiating a jog-walk program, stretching and moderate warm-up exercises (calisthenics) for 10 to 15 minutes followed by a continuous walk for 20 to 30 minutes on alternate days are recommended.

Participants can begin to increase their frequency of training to a daily basis after several weeks or months of conditioning. The point in time at which this increase in frequency can be accommodated properly is an individual matter and is dependent upon age and initial level of fitness. Generally, persons of older ages and lower fitness levels are more prone to musculoskeletal problems.

INTENSITY-DURATION. Although intensity and duration are separate entities in themselves, it is difficult to discuss intensity without mentioning its interaction with duration. As mentioned in Section 2, exercise regimens of lower intensity (less caloric expenditure) but with a longer duration period showed similar improvements to the higher intensity and shorter duration regimens; the total caloric expenditures were approximately equal for both programs. The caloric difference between running a mile in eight minutes and running a mile in nine minutes is minimal; therefore, running a little extra time or distance at the slower pace will offset the extra calories burned at the faster pace. The important concept is that as long as the intensity is above the minimal threshold level, and a certain amount of total work is completed in an exercise session (total calories), the manner in which it is accomplished can vary.

The above mentioned concept has important implications for exercise prescription for adults, and it should be remembered that low-intensity, longer-duration types of programs are generally recommended for beginners. This recommendation is particularly true for those showing a poor performance or presence of heart disease on their initial evaluation. The important point is to prescribe a regimen at a low intensity so that the participant can accomplish a sufficient amount of work. Initially the prescription may call for a moderate to brisk walk for 20 to 30 minutes duration.

Table 4.1 outlines a certain minimal threshold of intensity that is necessary for improving cardiorespiratory function. As was mentioned in Section 2 under research findings, programs of an intensity of less than 60 percent of maximum capacity will often produce improvement in persons with low initial levels of fitness. These persons generally will qualify for fitness classifications 1 or 2, as listed in Table 3.3. Special starter programs of less than 60 percent intensity are recommended for these individuals.

The training duration will vary from day to day and from activity to activity. The important factor is to design a program that meets the criteria for improving and maintaining a sufficient level of physical fitness, that is enjoyable (tolerable), and will fit into time demands.

It should be rewarding to the participant—preferably it should be fun.

The level of training intensity that can be tolerated will vary greatly depending on status of fitness and health, age, experience, and general ability. Long distance runners may tolerate two to three hours of continuous running at 80 to 90 percent of maximum capacity, but most beginners cannot perform a continuous effort at this level for more than a few minutes. For beginners to accomplish 20 to 30 minutes of continuous training, they must choose the proper intensity level. The proper intensity level for beginners will range from 60 to 70 percent of maximum capacity (brisk walking programs) to 70 to 80 percent of maximum capacity for jogging (the latter program is generally interspersed with bouts of walking, with intensity representing the peak intensity while jogging). Most persons in fitness categories 1 and 2 (Table 3.3) will start with a walking program, and those in categories 3 and above, with a combination walk-jog routine.

The walk-jog routine, or low-intensity, moderate-intensity periods of work if performing another mode of activity, will have a peak intensity of 85 to 90 percent of maximum capacity and a low intensity of 50 to 65 percent. The average intensity level will range between 70 and 80 percent of maximum capacity. Experience has shown that an intensity level of 50 to 60 percent of maximum can be tolerated comfortably for 20 to 30 minutes by most persons and can be classified as low to moderate work. Intensity levels ranging from 70 to 85 percent are considered as moderate work and those above 90 percent of maximum capacity as high-intensity work. The results of the initial stress test are important in placing the participant at a correct and safe level of intensity.

Upon initiating an endurance training regimen, most participants notice the training effect rather quickly. They usually experience the ability to perform more total work in subsequent exercise sessions. The increased total work is a result of the ability of the participant to increase the training duration and/or to tolerate a greater work intensity. The increased average intensity is a function of a higher peak intensity level and/or an increase in the ratio of high to low bouts of work. For example, a participant in a walk-jog routine can tolerate longer periods of jogging interspersed with shorter amounts of walking. As these adaptations to training occur, changes in the exercise prescription are recommended. Periodic reevaluations will help in determining a new status of physical fitness, enhance motivation, and facilitate proper exercise prescription.

How is a participant's exercise intensity determined and how can it be estimated during an exercise session? As mentioned in Section 3 under evaluation procedures, functional capacity is measured during a stress test. During the test, heart rate and in some cases oxygen consumption are measured or estimated. The exercise intensity is then estimated from a certain percentage of the functional maximum heart rate or oxygen uptake. The percentage of maximum at which a participant trains is called the target heart rate or target training load.

Heart rate and oxygen uptake have a linear relationship (see Figure 4.1). Thus, heart rate is considered an excellent means for estimating intensity of training. Because of the impracticality of routinely measuring oxygen uptake and the ease in monitoring heart rate, the heart rate standard is recommended for general use.

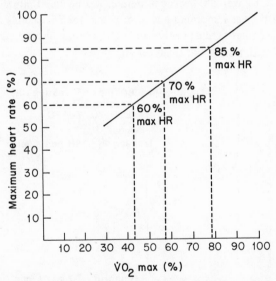

FIGURE 4.1. Figure shows the linear relationship between oxygen uptake and heart rate.

To make an accurate estimation of intensity of training or target training load, it is necessary to know both resting and maximum heart rates. Maximum heart rate can be determined by using the highest heart rate found on a maximum graded exercise test, after a difficult bout of endurance exercise, by subtracting one's age from 220, or by referring to Table 3.5. See Figure 4.2 for an example of calculating percent of maximum heart rate range. The first method of estimating maximum heart rate is preferred because there is considerable individual variation, and that heart rate is usually attained while qualified personnel are evaluating the performance of a participant. The second method is to count the heart rate after an all-out 12-minute run or similar endurance type field test (1.5-mile run). This type of test is not recommended for beginners or persons suspected of being coronary prone. The third and fourth methods of determining maximum heart rate are the least accurate, but may be used as a rough approximation. The inaccuracy of the third and fourth methods stems from the variability of maximum heart rate at any given age. For example, the maximum heart rate of a man 50 years of age averages approximately 170 beats per minute, but presumably healthy individuals may have rates from below 140 to over 200 beats per minute. Resting heart rate should be counted in the early morning just after rising, for 30 seconds while in a comfotable, quiet sitting position and before eating or smoking.

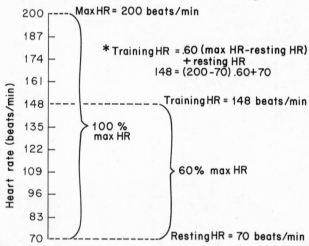

FIGURE 4.2. Karvonen formula for determination of training (target) heart rate. Also shown is an example of the calculation of training heart rate (*Karvonen et al).

Estimating exercise heart rate during training usually is accomplished by counting the pulse rate immediately after stopping by means of the palpation technique. This is performed by placing the tips of the first two fingers lightly on the carotid artery (adjacent to the voice box), on the radial artery (thumb side of the wrist), or the heel of the hand over the left side of the chest (at the apex of the heart) and by counting the pulsations. The pulse at the radial artery is generally more difficult to count after exercise and thus is not recommended. If using the carotid artery, caution must be taken not to apply too much pressure. Excessive pressure on the carotid artery may cause the heart rate to slow down by refex action. A few persons will not be able to count the pulse at any such site and will need to revert to the use of a stethoscope.

Heart rate begins to decelerate soon after cessation of exercising (usually after only 15 seconds); therefore, the count should begin as soon as possible. It is recommended that one count the pulse for 10 seconds and complete it within 15 seconds after cessation of exercise. Only two to four seconds are needed to position the hand or fingers properly and to feel the heart beat rhythm. Thus, by counting beats per 10 seconds, it is possible to complete the count within 15 seconds and to avoid errors resulting from the deceleration of the heart beat.

A wrist watch, wall clock, or stopwatch can be used for determining heart rate; however, a stopwatch will be the most accurate. The stopwatch facilitates starting the count more quickly as well as general counting accuracy. After establishing the heart rate rhythm, the count can start on a full beat with the first count being zero (can only start this way when using stopwatch). If the count does not end on an even beat, then one-half beat is added to the last full count. This counting detail is important with the 10 second technique because each one-beat error in counting results in a six beat per minute error.

Another heart rate counting procedure that can be used satisfactorily is to count beats per 15 seconds. This method has some advantages: counting the heart rate over a longer time span can reduce the errors in counting, and multiplying the counted value by four to get beats per minute is easier for the beginner. The disadvantage is the 5 to 10 percent error that may occur with the added counting time.

Each of the techniques requires some experimentation and practice to become proficient. Table 4.2 is a conversion chart for transforming raw heart rate data to beats per minute.

MODE OF ACTIVITY. Many different types of activities can provide adequate stimulation for improving cardiorespiratory function. Section 2 emphasized that the total energy cost of a program is an important factor and that as long as various activities are of sufficient intensity and duration, the training effect will occur. Also, activities of similar energy requirements will provide similar training effects. In choosing the proper mode of training, the participant should be familiar with the variety of activities that are available. Table 4.3 categorizes activities by their calorie cost (METS). An activity will vary in intensity depending on the enthusiasm of the participant as well as on the type of activity, for example, tennis singles or doubles; thus, a range of energy costs is listed in the table.

Generally, an activity that expends less than five calories per minute (<3.5 METS) is classified as "low" intensity and is not recommended for use in exercise regimens that are designed to develop cardiorespiratory fitness and weight reduction. An exception to this would be for a person with a functional capacity below 6 METS. These persons can often improve their functional capacity with low-intensity work, but should be encouraged to increase the duration of effort up to 60 minutes. Except for persons of extremely high or low functional capacities, activities that expend 5 to 10 calories per minute (4 to 8 METS) are considered of moderate intensity; activities from 10 to 14 calories per minute (8 to 12 METS), moderate to high intensity; and activities greater than 14 calories (12 METS), high intensity. These classifications are based upon exercising continuously for up to 60 minutes.

When choosing the proper activity, the participant should take into account level of fitness, health status, physical activity interests, availability of equipment and facilities, geographical location, and climate. The deconditioned adult should be involved initially in several weeks or months of moderate activity that does not require competition or extreme starting and stopping movements. Under these conditions, many participants tend to overdo it and become unduly stiff and sore, fatigued, or injured. Since the joints and muscular system are not adequately developed in a beginner to handle such demands, the participant is vulnerable to injury. The need to get in shape to play games is true in most cases. Persons whose screening tests have indicated cardiovascular problems should avoid highly competitive-type activities. *It is important not to exceed the safe limit of exercise.* The starter programs outlined later are recommended for beginners. (For more specific

TABLE 4.2. Conversion chart for transforming heart rate counted for 10 or 15 seconds to beats per minute

HEART RATE			
BEATS PER 10 SECONDS	BEATS PER MINUTE	BEATS PER 15 SECONDS	BEATS PER MINUTE
15	90	23	92
16	96	24	96
17	102	25	100
18	108	26	104
19	114	27	108
20	120	28	112
21	126	29	116
22	132	30	120
23	138	31	124
24	144	32	128
25	150	33	132
26	156	34	136
27	162	35	140
28	168	36	144
29	174	37	148
30	180	38	152
31	186	39	156
32	192	40	160
33	198	41	164
34	204	42	168
		43	172
		44	176
		45	180
		46	184
		47	188
		48	192
		49	196
		50	200
		51	204

TABLE 4.3. Energy cost of various activities[a]

ACTIVITY	CALORIES[b] (cal/min)	METS[c]	OXYGEN COST (ml/kg·min)
Archery	3.7-5	3-4	10.5-14
Backpacking	6-13.5	5-11	17.5-38.5
Badminton	5-11	4-9	14-31.5
Basketball			
Nongame	3.7-11	3-9	10.5-31.5
Game	8.5-15	7-12	24.5-42
Bed exercise (arm movement, supine or sitting)	1.1-2.5	1-2	3.5-7
Bicycling			
(pleasure or to work)	3.7-10	3-8	10.5-28
Bowling	2.5-5	2-4	7-14
Canoeing			
(rowing and kayaking)	3.7-10	3-8	10.5-28
Calisthenics	3.7-10	3-8	10.5-28
Dancing (social and square)	3.7-8.5	3-7	10.5-24.5
Fencing	7.5-12	6-10	21-35
Fishing			
(bank, boat, or ice)	2.5-5	2-4	7-14
(stream, wading)	6-7.5	5-6	17.5-21
Football (touch)	7.5-12	6-10	21-35
Golf			
(Using power cart)	2.5-3.7	2-3	7-10.5
(walking, carrying bag, or pulling cart)	5-8.5	4-7	14-24.5
Handball	10-15	8-12	28-42
Hiking (Cross-country)	3.7-8.5	3-7	10.5-24.5
Horseback riding	3.7-10	3-8	10.5-28
Horseshoe pitching	2.5-3.7	2-3	7-10.5
Hunting, walking			
Small game	3.7-8.5	3-7	10.5-24.5
Big game	3.7-17	3-14	10.5-49
Jogging (See Table 4.4)			
Mountain climbing	6-12	5-10	17.5-35
Paddleball (racquet)	10-15	8-12	28-42

Sailing	2.5-6	2-5	7-17.5
Scuba diving	6-12	5-10	17.5-35
Shuffleboard	2.5-3.7	2-3	7-10.5
Skating (ice or roller)	6-10	5-8	17.5-28
Skiing (snow)			
Downhill	6-10	5-8	17.5-28
Cross-country	7.5-15	6-12	21-42
Skiing (water)	6-8.5	5-7	17.5-24.5
Snow shoeing	8.5-17	7-14	24.5-49
Squash	10-15	8-12	28-42
Soccer	6-15	5-12	17.5-42
Softball	3.7-7.5	3-6	10.5-21
Stair-climbing	5-10	4-8	14-28
Swimming	5-10	4-8	14-28
Table tennis	3.7-6	3-5	10.5-17.5
Tennis	5-11	4-9	14-31.5
Volleyball	3.7-7.5	3-6	10.5-21
Walking (See Table 4.4)			

[a]Energy cost values based on an individual of 154 pounds of body weight (70 kg).
[b]Calorie: a unit of measure based upon heat production. One calorie equals approximately 200 milliliters of oxygen consumed.
[c]MET: basal oxygen requirement of the body sitting quietly. One MET equals 3.5 milliliters of oxygen per kilogram of body weight per minute.

information concerning cardiac rehabilitation, see Section 5.)

Participation in a variety of activities is recommended and can be accomplished by interchanging some of the various activities listed in Table 4.3. Choosing different activities tends to keep a participant interested in endurance exercise over a long-term period. For example, one might jog 30 minutes on Monday and Thursday and play handball or basketball on Tuesday and Friday. The important factor is for the person to participate in these activities frequently and with sufficient intensity and duration.

Regardless of the type of physical activity used in a training program, each exercise session should begin with a warm-up period and finish with a cool-down period. The warm-up period should be from 10 to 15 minutes in duration and include a combination of stretching (flexibility) and light-to-moderate muscular strength and endurance excercises. These warm-up exercises can be followed by five minutes of walking or slow jogging. Suggested stretching and muscular strength and endurance exercises are described later.

The cool-down period should allow adequate time for the various bodily processes to readjust to normal. The length of the cool-down period is dependent on the difficulty of the endurance training period, status of physical fitness, and environmental conditions. Persons in better physical condition recover more quickly from vigorous activity. Exercising in a hot and humid environment generally will lengthen the recovery period. The cool-down period normally will last from 5 to 10 minutes and can include a variety of activities such as slow jogging, walking, stretching, and light calisthenics.

Although the emphasis of this discussion was based upon the variety of activities available for developing and maintaining cardiorespiratory endurance, remember that this exercise is only a part of a total, well-rounded program. Endurance activities are of paramount importance, but adequate flexibility and muscular strength and muscular endurance add to a balanced physical fitness program.

TARGET HEART RATE FOR HIGH RISK AND CARDIAC PA-TIENTS. For exercise prescription, the target heart rate is the recommended training heart rate. It is based upon the results of the exercise tolerance test (functional capacity). As mentioned earlier, during a training program the training heart rate will vary from 60 (120 to 140 beats per minute) to 90 percent (170 to 190 beats per minute) of maximum heart rate range. It was also mentioned that the intensity will vary depending on the participant's *age, level of fitness, and status of health.* Although target heart rates should be generally established for all beginners, it is of particular importance to the *high risk* and *cardiac patient.* These persons generally have abnormal exercise test results or have a symptom limited test response, that is, the stress test was terminated as a result of contraindications to continue the test (severe chest discomfort or pain, too many irregular heart beats, ST depression of the ECG, etc.).

For these participants, not exceeding the target heart rate would be extremely important. Also, a target heart rate should be based at a level at which dangerous symptoms or signs are not present. For the beginning cardiac patient this should be 10 to 15 beats per minute below the symptom level. Once the cardiac or high risk patients have been in the program for several weeks, the target heart rate may be increased. Any increase in intensity would be based on the fact that the patient is stable and adapting well to the starter program. It is strongly recommended that the duration of training be increased sufficiently prior to any consideration of increased intensity (for more details in exercise prescription in cardiac patients see Section 5).

PROGRAMS FOR CARDIORESPIRATORY FITNESS AND WEIGHT CONTROL

Exercise programs that develop cardiorespiratory fitness and help individuals to reduce their body weight or fat are termed endurance exercises. Endurance exercises require a sustained effort, such as found in jogging, walking, bicycling, swimming, and vigorous game-type activities.

EXERCISE PRESCRIPTION FOR CARDIORESPIRATORY ENDURANCE AND WEIGHT CONTROL. As mentioned earlier, in order to prescribe exercise properly, it is necessary to know something about the person's health status and physical fitness level. After undergoing the physical fitness examination, a participant may be classified into one of eight categories of cardiorespiratory fitness. Table 3.3 shows the fitness classification scores achieved on various tests. In order to be classified into the good level of cardiorespiratory fitness, a person should have a functional capacity of approximately 42 to 45 milliliters per kilogram of body weight per minute of oxygen uptake (12 to 13 METS). Therefore, knowing the initial level of cardiorespiratory fitness will help guide the participant into the correct program.

The exercise prescription usually has three stages of progression: starter, slow progression, and maintenance (see Figure 4.3). The initial stage of training is classified as a starter program. In this phase the exercise intensity is low and includes a lot of stretching and light calisthenics. The purpose at this stage of the program is to introduce one to exercise at a low level and to allow time to adapt properly to the initial weeks of training. If this phase is introduced correctly, the participant will experience a minimum of muscle soreness and can avoid debilitating injuries or discomfort of the knee, shin, ankle, or foot. The latter injuries are common in the initial stages of a jogging program, but can be avoided if the participant takes some preliminary precautions, such as a good starter program, use of good training shoes,

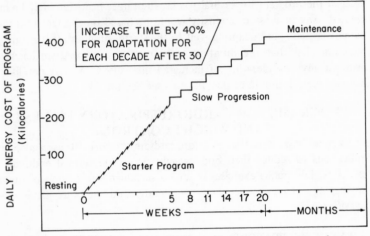

FIGURE 4.3 Diagramatic view of exercise prescription in relation to progression in training.

and proper warm-up and conditioning of the legs. Avoiding sharp turns and extremely hard running surfaces are also important safeguards (See Section 7 for more detail).

The duration of the starter program is usually from four to six weeks, but is dependent on the adaptation of the participant to the program. For example, a person who is classified in a poor or fair fitness level may spend as many as 6 to 10 weeks in a starter program, but a participant scoring in the good to excellent categories may not need to participate in a starter program.

The slow progression stage of training differs from the starter phase in that the participant is progressed at a more rapid rate. During this stage, the duration or intensity are increased rather consistently every two to three weeks. How well the person adapts to the present level of training dictates the frequency and magnitude of progression. As a general rule, the older the participant and the lower the initial fitness level, the longer one takes to adapt and progress in a training regimen. The adaptation to the training load takes approximately 40 percent longer for each decade in life after age 30. That is, if the progression in distance run is every two weeks for men of 30 to 39 years, then the interval may be three weeks for those of 40 to 49 years and four weeks for the 50 to 59 year old group.

The maintenance stage of prescription usually occurs after six months to a year of training. At this stage, the participant has reached a satisfactory level of cardiorespiratory fitness and may be no longer interested in increasing the training load. At this point further development is usually minimal, but continuing the same workout schedule (the number of miles or minutes trained per week) enables one to maintain fitness.

GENERAL GUIDELINES FOR GETTING STARTED. In designing an exercise regimen one must select activities that can be performed on a regular basis. Generally, game-type activities are not recommended in the early stages of training. Prior to becoming involved in game-type activities whereby running will be encountered, fast walking or walk-jog programs are recommended.

Table 4.3 lists the energy cost of a variety of activities commonly used in recreation and endurance fitness programs. The activities are quantified in terms of calories per minute, METS, and oxygen cost. These values indicate the relative intensity of the effort. To get the total effect of the programs, one must determine the intensity level and multiply this by the total number of minutes of participation. Because games are not played continuously with an even amount of effort (fuel supply), some approximation will have to be made to get the intensity level for game-type activities. Intensity is dependent on how hard the game is played. If in doubt use the average value listed in Table 4.3. For example, if handball is played for 45 minutes, then the intensity in calories (12.5 calories per minute) would be multiplied by the minutes played (45) to get the total calorie expenditure (562.5). The important point here is that the participant counts only the time that was used in participation. Rest breaks and standing around do not count.

The energy cost of running and walking is listed in Table 4.4. An endurance training program can be designed from Table 4.4 but, because of the difficulty of knowing the proper pace or sequence of progression, several programs are outlined in Tables 4.6 to 4.16. The programs include walking and running routines and are designed relative to various levels of fitness.

Although walking and running can be done in a variety of settings such as running tracks, roads, parks, and so on, the course should be a measured distance. This can be accomplished by the use of an odometer from an automobile or bicycle, or use of a measured track. Train-

TABLE 4.4. Energy cost of walking and running[a]

ACTIVITY	CALORIES[b] (Cal/min)	METS[c]
Walking	2.5	2.0
	3.0	2.5
	3.7	3.0
	6.0	5.0
	8.5	7.0
	11.0	9.0
	4.2	3.5
	7.5	5.9
	10.0	8.3
	13.0	10.7
	4.9	4.0
	5.5	4.6
	9.0	7.3
	12.0	10.0
	15.6	12.8
	7.0	5.7
	8.3	6.9
Running	10.1	8.3
	12.0	10.0
	14.0	11.5
	15.6	12.8
	17.5	14.2
	19.6	16.0
	21.7	17.7
	24.5	20.0

[a]Energy cost values based on an individual of 154 pounds of body weight (70 kg).
[b]Calorie: a unit of measure based upon heat production. One calorie equals 200 milliliters of oxygen consumed.
[c]Met: basal oxygen requirement of the body sitting quietly. One MET equals 3.5 milliliters of oxygen per kilogram of body weight.

| OXYGEN COST (ml/kg·min) | SPEED | | GRADE |
	MPH	MIN/MILE (min:sec)	(%)
7	2.0	30:00	0
8.7	2.5	24:00	0
10.5	3.0	20:00	0
17.5	3.0	20:00	5
24.5	3.0	20:00	10
31.5	3.0	20:00	15
12.3	3.5	17:08	0
21	3.5	17:08	5
29	3.5	17:08	10
37.5	3.5	17:08	15
14	3.75	16:00	0
16.1	4.0	15:00	0
25.6	4.0	15:00	5
35	4.0	15:00	10
44.8	4.0	15:00	15
20	4.5	13:20	0
24	5.0	12:00	0
29	5.5	10:55	0
35	6.0	10:00	0
40.3	7.0	8:35	0
44.8	8.0	7:30	0
49.7	9.0	6:40	0
56	10.0	6:00	0
62	11.0	5:30	0
70	12.0	5:00	0

Table 4.5. Pacing chart for walking and running program conducted on track measured in 110-yard increments

PACE			PACE			PACE		
110 yd (sec)	440 yd (min:sec)	mph	110 yd (sec)	440 yd (min:sec)	mph	110 yd (sec)	440 yd (min:sec)	mph
18	1:12	12.5	38	2:32	5.9	58	3:52	3.9
19	1:16	11.8	39	2:36	5.8	59	3:56	3.8
20	1:20	11.2	40	2:40	5.6	60	4:00	3.7
21	1:24	10.7	41	2:44	5.5	61	4:04	3.7
22	1:28	10.2	42	2:48	5.4	62	4:08	3.6
23	1:32	9.8	43	2:52	5.2	63	4:12	3.6
24	1:36	9.4	44	2:56	5.1	64	4:16	3.5
25	1:40	9.0	45	3:00	5.0	65	4:20	3.5
26	1:44	8.6	46	3:04	4.9	66	4:24	3.4
27	1:48	8.3	47	3:08	4.8	67	4:28	3.4
28	1:52	8.0	48	3:12	4.7	68	4:32	3.3
29	1:56	7.7	49	3:16	4.6	69	4:36	3.3
30	2:00	7.5	50	3:20	4.5	70	4:40	3.2
31	2:04	7.3	51	3:24	4.4	71	4:44	3.2
32	2:08	7.0	52	3:28	4.3	72	4:48	3.1
33	2:12	6.8	53	3:32	4.2	73	4:52	3.1
34	2:16	6.6	54	3:36	4.2	74	4:56	3.0
35	2:20	6.4	55	3:40	4.1	75	5:00	3.0
36	2:24	6.2	56	3:44	4.0	76	5:04	2.9
37	2:28	6.1	57	3:48	3.9	77	5:08	2.9

TABLE 4.6. Six-week starter programs for persons in fitness categories 1 and 2[a]

PROGRAM	WEEK	PACE (mph)	DISTANCE (miles)	TIME (min:sec)	CALORIES
A	1	3.0	1.5	36:00	133
	2	3.5	1.5	25:42	107
	3	3.5	2.0	34:16	143
	4	3.5	2.0	34:16	143
	5	3.5	2.5	42:50	179
	6	3.5	2.5	42:50	179
B	1	3.5	2.0	34:16	143
	2	3.5	2.0	34:16	143
	3	4.0	2.0	30:00	165
	4	4.0	2.0	30:00	165
	5	4.0	2.5	37:50	206
	6	4.0	2.5	37:50	206

[a]Programs based upon level walking at sea level and in an average climatic condition (temperature and humidity).

TABLE 4.7. Six-week starter program for persons in fitness category 3[a]

| PROGRAM | WEEK | WALK | | | RUN | |
		PACE (mph)	DISTANCE (yd)	TIME (sec)	PACE (mph)	DISTANCE (yd)
A	1	3.75	110	60	5.5	110
	2	3.75	110	60	5.5	110
	3	3.75	110	60	5.5	220
	4	3.75	110	60	5.5	220
	5	3.75	110	60	5.5	330
	6	3.75	110	60	5.5	330
B	1	3.75	110	60	6.4	110
	2	3.75	110	60	6.4	110
	3	3.75	110	60	6.4	220
	4	3.75	110	60	6.4	220
	5	3.75	110	60	6.4	330
	6	3.75	110	60	6.4	330

[a] Programs based upon level walking at sea level and in an average climatic condition (temperature and humidity).

RUN	REPETITIONS				
TIME (min:sec)	WALK	RUN	TIME (min:sec)	CALORIES	TOTAL MILES
:41	16	16	26:56	188.8	2.0
:41	16	16	26:56	188.8	2.0
1:22	11	11	26:02	205.7	2.0
1:22	11	11	26:02	205.7	2.0
2:03	8	8	24:24	204.8	2.0
2:03	8	8	24:24	204.8	2.0
:35	16	16	25:20	197.8	2.0
:35	16	16	25:20	197.8	2.0
1:10	11	11	23:50	218.0	2.0
1:10	12	12	26:00	238.0	2.25
1:45	9	9	24:45	245.7	2.25
1:45	9	9	24:45	245.7	2.25

TABLE 4.8. Six-week starter program for persons in fitness category 4[a]

PROGRAM	WEEK	WALK			RUN	
		PACE (mph)	DISTANCE (yd)	TIME (sec)	PACE (mph)	DISTANCE (yd)
A	1	3.75	110	60	6.8	220
	2	3.75	110	60	6.8	220
	3	3.75	110	60	6.8	330
	4	3.75	110	60	6.8	330
	5	3.75	110	60	6.8	440
	6	3.75	110	60	6.8	440
B	1	3.75	110	60	7.5	220
	2	3.75	110	60	7.5	220
	3	3.75	110	60	7.5	330
	4	3.75	110	60	7.5	330
	5	3.75	110	60	7.5	440
	6	3.75	110	60	7.5	440

[a] Programs based upon level walking at sea level and in an average climatic condition (temperature and humidity).

RUN TIME (min:sec)	REPETITIONS WALK	RUN	TIME (min:sec)	CALORIES	TOTAL MILES
1:06	11	11	23:06	218.5	2.0
1:06	11	11	23:06	218.5	2.0
1:39	8	8	22:12	218.7	2.0
1:39	9	9	23:51	246.1	2.25
2:12	8	8	23:24	248.6	2.25
2:12	8	8	25:36	278.6	2.25
1:00	12	12	24:00	236.4	2.25
1:00	12	12	24:00	236.4	2.25
1:30	9	9	22:30	243.9	2.25
1:30	10	10	25.00	271.0	2.25
2:00	8	8	24:00	276.0	2.25
2:00	8	8	24:00	276.0	2.25

TABLE 4.9. Six-week starter program for persons in fitness category 5[a]

| PROGRAM | WEEK | WALK | | | RUN | |
		PACE (mph)	DISTANCE (yd)	TIME (sec)	PACE (mph)	DISTANCE (yd)
A	1	3.75	110	60	7.5	330
	2	3.75	110	60	7.5	330
	3	3.75	110	60	7.5	440
	4	3.75	110	60	7.5	550
	5	3.75	110	60	7.5	660
	6	3.75	110	60	7.5	880
B	1	3.75	110	60	8.0	330
	2	3.75	110	60	8.0	330
	3	3.75	110	60	8.0	440
	4	3.75	110	60	8.0	550
	5	3.75	110	60	8.0	660
	6	3.75	110	60	8.0	880

[a] Programs based upon level walking at sea level and in an average climatic condition (temperature and humidity).

RUN TIME (min:sec)	REPETITIONS		TIME (min:sec)	CALORIES	TOTAL MILES
	WALK	RUN			
1:30	9	9	22:30	243.9	2.25
1:30	9	9	22:30	243.9	2.25
2:00	8	8	24:00	276.0	2.5
2:30	7	7	24:30	293.3	2.63
3:00	6	6	24:00	295.8	2.65
4:00	5	5	25:00	320.5	2.81
1.24	9	9	21.36	240.7	2.25
1:24	9	9	21:36	240.7	2.25
1:52	8	8	22:56	272.1	2.5
2:20	7	7	23:20	289.1	2.63
2:48	6	6	22:48	291.5	2.63
3:16	5	6	24:37	330.5	3.3

TABLE 4.10. Twenty-week walking program for fitness category 1[a]

WEEK	PACE (mph)	DISTANCE (miles)	TIME (min:sec)	CALORIES
1,2	3.75	2.5	40:00	196
3-5	3.75	2.75	44:00	215.6
6-8	4.0	2.75	41:15	226.9
9-12	4.0	3.0	45:00	247.5
13-16	4.25	3.0	42:21	262.0
16-20	4.25	3.25	45:53	285.4

[a]Programs based upon level walking at sea level and in an average climatic condition (temperature and humidity).

ing on an oval track can get boring over a long period of time, but if available, is a good way of getting started. Tracks generally have a smooth running surface and are of a known distance.

Table 4.5 will help in determining pace for walking and running programs. Speeds range from a slow walk (2.9 miles per hour) to a fast run (12.5 miles per hour). To aid in pacing, reference points of 110 or 440 yards are helpful. If carrying a stopwatch or wristwatch with a 60 second sweep hand, pace can be kept very accurately during the entire training program. Monitoring of the program by pace and heart rate response will help as a guide to proper initiation and progression of the training regimen.

Generally persons scoring in fitness categories 1 and 2 should begin their endurance training by walking. The walk should be at a comfortable but brisk pace. The initial speed may range from 3.0 to 4.0 miles per hour. Distance (or time) will be approximately one-and-one-half to two miles (30 to 40 minutes). The reason behind this combination of walking speed and distance is to get the participant started at a comfortable pace and at the same time keeping the distance long enough so that one can begin to get an endurance training effect.

Even though the calorie cost of this regimen is low (125 to 150 calories), it will allow time for adaptation of most bodily systems and parts. Do not be concerned about not working hard enough. Time, with proper progression and adaptation, will eventually lead to the higher, more demanding levels of training. Table 4.6 outlines two examples of six-week starter programs for walking, with Program A being recommended for persons in fitness category 1 and Program B for persons in fitness category 2. See Table 3.3 for placement into proper fitness category.

If one of the two examples of starter programs listed in Table 4.6 is too easy or difficult then make an on-the-spot change in the program. Remember, the exercise prescription should be individualized. A satisfactory modification can usually be made by changing the speed or distance slightly (Tables 4.4 and 4.5).

The programs listed here are based upon running or walking on a relatively flat surface, at sea level, and in an average climatic condition (temperature and humidity). Further program modifications will have to be taken into account when persons are exercising in moderate to extreme environmental conditions. Section 7 will discuss these modifications in more detail.

Once the participant has completed the six-week starter program, then the walking program listed in Tables 4.10 and 4.11 or the combination walk-jog program outlined in Table 4.7 can be initiated. The starter program outlined in Table 4.7 is recommended for persons scoring in fitness category 3. Tables 4.8 and 4.9 show suggested starter programs for persons scoring in fitness categories 4 and 5. Normally participants scoring in fitness categories above 50 milliliters per kilogram of body weight per minute of oxygen uptake (14 METS) are considered in excellent cardiorespiratory fitness and do not require a special starter program. Persons scoring in the excellent categories of fitness who have not been exercising on a regular basis should begin with the program outlined in Table 4.16.

MAINTENANCE PROGRAMS FOR CARDIORESPIRATORY FITNESS AND WEIGHT CONTROL. Upon completion of the 6-week starter and 20-week training programs outlined in Tables 4.6 to 4.16, a substantial improvement in fitness should have been attained. To maintain fitness, a specific program should be designed that will be similar in caloric cost to the initial program and also satisfy the needs of the participant over a long time-span. For many, walking and jogging may become boring and thus variety should be introduced into their program. The important point is that participation in activities that are enjoyed is more likely to be continued.

Check over the list of activities in Table 4.3 to see which ones best meet your interest and can still give the caloric consumption necessary

TABLE 4.11. Twenty-week walking-jogging program for fitness category 2[a]

		WALK			RUN	
WEEK	PACE (mph)	DISTANCE	TIME (min:sec)	PACE (mph)	DISTANCE (yd)	TIME (min:sec)
1,2	4.0	2.75 mi	41:15			
3,4	4.25	2.75 mi	38:50			
5,6	4.25	3.0 mi	42:21			
7,8	4.5	3.0 mi	40:00			
9,10	4.5	3.25 mi	43:20			
11,12	4.0	110 yd	1:00	4.75	220	1:35
13,14	4.0	110 yd	1:00	4.75	330	2:22
15,16	4.0	110 yd	1:00	4.75	440	3:10
17,18	4.0	110 yd	1:00	5.0	330	2:15
19,20	4.0	110 yd	1:00	5.0	440	3:00

[a] Programs based upon level walking at sea level and in an average climatic condition (temperature and humidity).
[b] Ten walk, 11 run.

REPETITIONS	TOTAL TIME (min:sec)	CALORIES	TOTAL MILES
1	41:15	226.9	
1	38:50	241.5	
1	42:21	262.0	
1	40:00	280.0	
1	43:20	303.2	
18	46:26	316.6	3.375
13	43:49	307.2	3.25
10/11[b]	44:50	321.4	3.375
13	42:15	314.3	3.25
10/11[b]	43:00	328.9	3.375

TABLE 4.12. Twenty-week walk-jog, jogging program for fitness category 3A[a]

	WALK			RUN		
WEEK	**PACE (mph)**	**DISTANCE (yd)**	**TIME (sec)**	**PACE (mph)**	**DISTANCE (yd:mi)**	**TIME (min:sec)**
1, 2	3.75	110	60	5.6	440:1/4	2:41
3, 4	3.75	110	60	5.6	660:	4:01
5, 6	3.75	110	60	5.6	880:1/2	5:22
7, 8	3.75	110	60	5.6	1320:3/4	8:02
					550:	3:20
9, 10	3.75	110	60	5.6	1760:1	10:42
11, 12	3.75	110	60	5.6	:1 1/4	13:20
					:1/2	5:22
13, 14	3.75	110	60	5.6	:1 1/2	16:04
15, 16	3.75	110	60	5.6	:2	21:24
					:1	10:42
17, 18	3.75	110		5.6	:2 1/2	26:47
					:1/2	5:22
19, 20				5.6	:3	32:08

[a] Programs based upon level walking at sea level and in an average climatic condition (temperature and humidity).

REPETITIONS	TOTAL TIME (min:sec)	CALORIES	TOTAL MILES
8	29:26	259.9	2.5
6	30:06	277.6	2.63
5	31:47	300.4	2.81
3	30:27	297.2	2.75
1			
3	35:08	345.7	3.19
2	34:08	340.6	3.13
1			
2	34:08	340.8	3.13
1	33:08	335.5	3.06
1			
1	33:09	336.0	3.06
1			
1	32:08	331.0	3.00

TABLE 4.13. Twenty-week walk-jog, jogging program for fitness category 3B[a]

	WALK			RUN		
WEEK	PACE (mph)	DISTANCE (yd)	TIME (sec)	PACE (mph)	DISTANCE (yd:mi)	TIME (min:sec)
1, 2	3.75	110	60	6.4	440:1/4	2:20
3, 4	3.75	110	60	6.4	660:	3:30
5, 6	3.75	110	60	6.4	880:1/2	4:20
7, 8	3.75	110	60	6.4	1320:3/4	7:00
					550:	2:55
9, 10	3.75	110	60	6.4	1760:1	9:24
11, 12	3.75	110	60	6.4	:1 1/4	11:44
					:1/2	4:20
13, 14	3.75	110	60	6.4	:1 1/2	13:44
15, 16	3.75	110	60	6.4	:2	18:48
					:1	9:24
17, 18	3.75	110	60	6.4	:2 1/2	23:08
					:1/2	4:20
19, 20				6.4	:3	28:12

[a] Programs based upon level walking at sea level and in an average climatic condition (temperature and humidity).

REPETITIONS	TOTAL TIME (min:sec)	CALORIES	TOTAL MILES
8	26:40	278.2	2.5
6	27:00	298.2	2.63
5	26:40	301.7	2.81
3	26:55	320.7	2.75
1			
3	29:12	365.8	3.19
2	28:48	360.7	3.13
1			
2	28:28	356.5	3.13
1	29:12	365.8	3.06
1			
1	28:28	356.4	3.06
1			
1	28:12	361.0	3.00

TABLE 4.14. Twenty-week walk-jog, jogging program for fitness category 4A[a]

| | WALK | | | RUN | | |
WEEK	PACE (mph)	DISTANCE (yd)	TIME (sec)	PACE (mph)	DISTANCE (yd:mi)	TIME (min:sec)
1, 2	3.75	110	60	6.8	660:	3:18
3, 4	3.75	110	60	6.8	880:1/2	4:24
5, 6	3.75	110	60	6.8	1320:3/4	6:36
					550:	2:45
7, 8	3.75	110	60	6.8	1760:1	8:48
9, 10	3.75	110	60	6.8	:1 1/4	11:00
					:1/2	4:24
11, 12	3.75	110	60	6.8	:1 1/2	13:12
13, 14	3.75	110	60	6.8	:2	17:36
					:1 1/4	11:00
15, 16	3.75	110	60	6.8	:2 1/2	22:00
					:3/4	6:36
17, 18	3.75	110	60	6.8	:3 1/4	28:36
19, 20				6.8	:3 1/2	30:48

[a] Programs based upon level walking at sea level and in an average climatic condition (temperature and humidity).

REPETITIONS	TOTAL TIME (min:sec)	CALORIES	TOTAL MILES
6	25:48	298.7	2.63
5	27:00	323.7	2.81
3	25:33	321.4	2.75
1			
3	29:24	373.7	3.19
2	28:24	368.8	3.13
1			
2	28:24	368.8	3.13
1	29:36	393.9	3.31
1			
1	29:36	393.9	3.31
1			
1	28:36	389.0	3.25
1	30:48	418.9	3.5

TABLE 4.15. Twenty-week walk-jog, jogging program for fitness category 4B[a]

WEEK	WALK			RUN		
	PACE (mph)	DISTANCE (yd)	TIME (sec)	PACE (mph)	DISTANCE (yd:mi)	TIME (min:sec)
1, 2	3.75	110	60	7.5	660:	3:00
3, 4	3.75	110	60	7.5	880:1/2	4:00
5, 6	3.75	110	60	7.5	1320:3/4	6:00
					550:	2:30
7, 8	3.75	110	60	7.5	1760:1	8:00
9, 10	3.75	110	60	7.5	:1 1/4	10:00
					:1/2	4:00
11, 12	3.75	110	60	7.5	:1 1/2	12:00
13, 14	3.75	110	60	7.5	:2	16:00
					:1 1/4	10:00
15, 16	3.75	110	60	7.5	:2 1/2	20:00
					:3/4	6:00
17, 18				7.5	:3 1/4	26:00
19, 20				7.5	:3 1/2	28:00

[a] Programs based upon level walking at sea level and in an average climatic condition (temperature and humidity).

REPETITIONS	TOTAL TIME (min:sec)	CALORIES	TOTAL MILES
6	24:00	295.8	2.63
5	25:00	320.5	2.81
3	23:00	318.1	2.75
1			
3	27:00	369.9	3.19
2	26:00	365.0	3.13
1			
2	26:00	365.0	3.13
1	27:00	389.7	3.31
1			
1	27.00	389.7	3.31
1			
1	26:00	384.8	3.25
1	28:00	414.4	3.50

TABLE 4.16. Twenty-week walk-jog, jogging program for fitness category 5[a]

WEEK	WALK			RUN		
	PACE (mph)	DISTANCE (yd)	TIME (sec)	PACE (mph)	DISTANCE (yd:mi)	TIME (min:sec)
1, 2	3.75	110	60	7.5	880:1/2	4:00
3, 4	3.75	110	60	7.5	1320:3/4	6:00
5, 6	3.75	110	60	7.5	1760:1	8:00
					880:1/2	4:00
7, 8	3.75	110	60	7.5	:1 1/2	12:00
					:1/2	4:00
9, 10	3.75	110	60	7.5	:2	16:00
					:1 1/2	12:00
11, 12				7.5	:3	24:00
13, 14				7.5	:3 1/2	28:00
15, 16				7.5	:4	32:00
17, 18				7.7	:4	31:10
19, 20				8.0	:4	30:00

[a] Programs based upon level walking at sea level and in an average climatic condition (temperature and humidity).

REPETITIONS	TOTAL TIME (min:sec)	CALORIES	TOTAL MILES
6	30:00	384.6	3.38
4	28:00	374.8	3.25
3	31:00	429.1	3.69
1			
2	30:00	424.2	3.63
1			
1	30:00	424.2	3.56
1			
1	24:00	355.0	3.0
1	28:00	414.8	3.3
1	32:00	473.6	4.0
1	31:10	470.6	4.0
1	30:00	468.0	4.0

for maintenance. Fitness is not stored but must be practiced continually. The guidelines for frequency, intensity, and duration of training do not change and should be taken into consideration when selecting activities for participation.

If goals have not been met or further development is required, then added caloric expenditure is needed. For example, since ideal weight may not be attained in a 20-week program, the program design should increase caloric output. Usually added frequency of training of up to five or six days per week will greatly increase the total energy expenditure. The addition of one extra 400-calorie workout per week to the training regimen should remove 1 pound of fat every nine weeks. If this is matched by a similar reduction in food intake, it will amount to a reduction of 12 pounds in a year.

PROGRAMS FOR MUSCULAR STRENGTH AND ENDURANCE, AND FLEXIBILITY

As described in Section 2, muscular strength and endurance are developed by using the overload principle; that is, applying more tension on the muscle than is normally used. Muscular strength is best developed by using heavy weights (maximum or near maximum tension applied) with few repetitions and muscular endurance by using lighter loads along with a greater number of repetitions. To some extent both strength and endurance can be developed under each condition, but each system favors a more specific type of development.

Muscular strength and endurance can be developed by means of either isometric (static), isotonic (going through the full range of motion), or isokinetic exercise (see Section 2 for further explanation). Although each type of training has its strong and weak points, isotonic and isokinetic exercises are recommended for the development and maintenance of muscular strength and endurance. Isotonic exercises should be rhythmical, follow through the full range of motion, and not impede normal forced breathing. Lifting heavy weights impedes blood circulation and breathing and can be potentially dangerous for persons with high blood pressure, coronary heart disease, and other circulatory problems. Therefore, the use of lighter weights is recommended.

It has already been stated that the emphasis of the exercise prescription should be based on a good endurance conditioning program that is supplemented by an exercise routine to develop and maintain muscular strength, endurance, and flexibility. It is felt that this type of training program best meets the interests and needs of the adult population. Therefore, as an adjunct to the previously described aerobics program, a series of exercises to develop and maintain muscular strength, endurance, and flexibility for most of the major muscle groups of the body are outlined.

The exercise routines are divided into the following categories: upper body, trunk, and lower back stretching (1 through 6); leg stretching (7 through 12); and muscular strength and endurance (12 through 20). Many of the exercises have several options from which to choose. In the first two categories (stretching exercises), some of the alternate exercises are more advanced and should be used only after the original exercise has been mastered. The muscular strength and endurance exercises offer options depending on whether or not weight training equipment is available.

The stretching exercises should be included as part of the warm-up routine prior to starting the aerobics phase of the program. The muscular strength and endurance routine can be used either after the stretching routine or after the aerobic phase.

Before starting the aforementioned routines one should make sure he or she is familiar with the described starting position, movement, and suggested repetitions. The training load has been designed to give the participant a moderate amount of muscular strength and endurance. We feel that this is the safest and most sensible manner to approach flexibility, and muscular strength and endurance training.

To help avoid muscle soreness in weight training exercises, the starting weight should be light (approximately 50% of the maximum that can be lifted in one repetition). After a few weeks of training, 60 to 70 percent of maximum can be attained. As soon as the required number of repetitions can be easily managed, more weight can be added. This is usually accomplished by adding 5 pounds of weight for arm and 10 pounds for leg exercises. For those participants who want to place more emphasis on strength development, a different training load and added sets would be necessary. The texts by Rasch or Hooks are recommended for more advanced weight training programs.

UPPER BODY, TRUNK, AND LOWER BACK
STRETCHING EXERCISES

1. TRUNK ROTATION

Purpose:	To stretch muscles in the back, sides, and shoulder girdle.
Starting Position:	Stand astride with feet pointed forward; raise arms to shoulder level. May use bar to increase stretch to the deltoid muscle and waist.
Movement:	Twist trunk to the right; avoid lifting heels. Repeat 3 to 4 times before twisting to left side.
Repetitions:	10

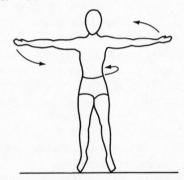

2. DOUBLE ARM CIRCLES AND TOE RAISES

Purpose:	To stretch muscles of the shoulder girdle and to strengthen muscles of the feet.
Starting Position:	Stand with feet about 12 inches apart and arms at sides.
Movement:	Swing arms upward and around, making large circles. As arms are raised and crossed overhead, rise on toes.
Repetitions:	10 to 15

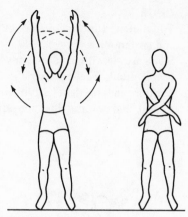

3a. FORWARD BEND

  Purpose: To stretch muscles of the buttocks and posterior leg.

Starting Position: Stand astride with hands on hips.

  Movement: Slowly bend forward to a 90-degree angle; return slowly to starting position; keep back flat.

Repetitions: 10

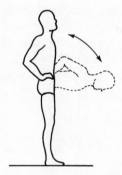

3b. ABDOMINAL CHURN

Purpose:	To stretch muscles of the buttocks, abdomen, and posterior leg.
Starting Position:	Stand astride with hands on hips.
Movement:	Lower trunk sideward to left; rotate to forward position and to right; return to upright position. Repeat and reverse direction after two rotations.
Repetitions:	5 to 8

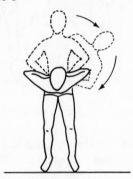

3c. BAR HANG

Purpose:	To stretch muscles of arms, shoulders, back, trunk, hips, and pelvic regions. Good general body stretcher.
Starting Position:	Hang from bar with arms straight.
Repetitions:	1 for up to 60 seconds

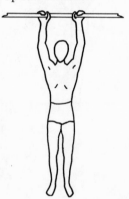

4. SHOULDER AND CHEST STRETCH

Purpose: To stretch muscles of the chest and shoulders.

Starting Position: Stand astride or kneel with arms at shoulder level and elbows bent.

Movement: Slowly force elbows backward and return to starting position.

Repetitions: 10 to 15

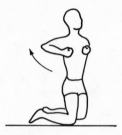

5a. LOWER BACK STRETCH

Purpose: To stretch muscles in the lower back.

Starting Position: Crouch on hands and knees.

Movement: Slowly rock back until buttocks touch heels; emphasize rounding back; return to starting position.

Repetitions: 10

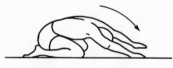

5b. ALTERNATE LOWER BACK STRETCH

Purpose: To stretch muscles in the lower back and buttocks.

Starting Position: Lie on back with the legs extended or stand erect.

Movement: Lift and bend one leg; grasp the knee and keep the opposite leg flat; pull knee to chest. Repeat with alternate leg.

Repetitions: 10

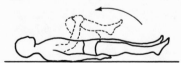

5c. ADVANCED LOWER BACK AND HAMSTRING STRETCH

Purpose:	To stretch muscles of the lower back and hamstring muscles.
Starting Position:	Lie on back with legs bent.
Movement:	Keep knees together and slowly bring them over the head; straighten the legs and touch the toes to the floor; return to starting position.
Repetitions:	5 to 10

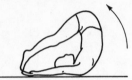

6. INVERTED STRETCH

Purpose:	To stretch and strengthen the anterior hip, buttocks, and abdominal muscles.
Starting Position:	Sit with arms at side.
Movement:	Support body with heels and arms and raise trunk as high as possible.
Repetitions:	10

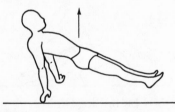

7a. FRONT LEG STRETCH

Purpose:	To stretch the muscles in the anterior leg.
Starting Position:	Kneel with tops of ankles and feet flat on the ground.
Movement:	Lean backward slowly; keep the back straight; maintain tension on muscles for 30 to 60 seconds.
Repetitions:	1 to 2

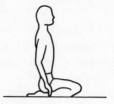

7b. FRONT LEG STRETCH

Purpose:	To stretch the muscles of the anterior thigh and hip.
Starting Position:	Lie on the ground with face down or stand erect.
Movement:	Pull the ankle to the hip slowly; hold for three seconds and release the ankle.Use same procedure for other side.
Note:	If difficulty is encountered in assuming starting position, ask for assistance.
Repetitions:	5 to 10

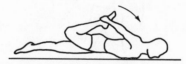

7c. ADVANCED FRONT LEG STRETCH

Purpose:	To stretch the muscles of the anterior thigh and leg.
Starting Position:	Kneel with feet turned outward.
Movement:	Lean backward slowly; put constant tension on muscles; use arms to control the movement; hold backward position for 30 to 60 seconds.
Repetitions:	1 to 2

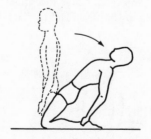

8. SIDE STRETCH

Purpose: To stretch the medial muscles of the thigh and the lateral muscles of the trunk and thorax.

Starting Position: Stand erect with one arm extended upward and the other relaxed at the side; place feet apart at more than shoulder width.

Movement: Bend trunk directly to the right with the left arm stretching overhead; keep both feet flat. Use same procedure for other side.

Repetitions: 5 to 10

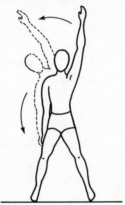

9. GROIN STRETCH

Purpose: To stretch the groin muscles.

Starting Position: Sit with knees bent outward and the bottoms of feet together.

Movement: Grasp ankles and pull the upper body as close as possible to the feet. Hold stretch for 30 to 60 seconds.

Repetitions: 1 to 2

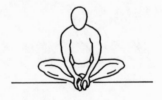

10. HAMSTRING STRETCH

Purpose:	To stretch the muscles in the posterior leg and thigh.
Starting Position:	Sit on ground with one leg extended straight forward; place the other leg forward with the knee bent and the sole touching the inner thigh of the extended leg.
Movement:	Bend forward and attempt to touch the head to the knee; hold stretch for 30 to 60 seconds. Repeat with other leg.
Repetitions:	1 to 2

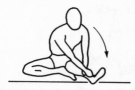

11a. CALF STRETCHER

Purpose:	To stretch the posterior leg and ankle muscles.
Starting Position:	Stand in forward stride position with the forward knee partially flexed and the rear leg fully extended; keep feet pointed forward and heels flat on the ground.
Movement:	Lean trunk forward until a continuous stretch occurs in the rear calf; hold stretch for 30 to 60 seconds. Repeat with other leg.
Repetitions:	1 to 2

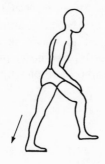

11*b*. CALF STRETCHER

Purpose:	To stretch the posterior leg muscles.
Starting Position:	Stand in upright position with the balls of the feet on the edge of a step.
Movement:	Slowly lower heels and hold for 30 to 60 seconds; raise heels and rise on toes.
Repetitions:	1 to 2

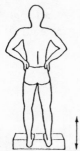

MUSCULAR STRENGTH AND ENDURANCE EXERCISES

Two options will be illustrated for each of the following routines. The first option (*a*) will utilize weights; the second (*b*) stresses the same muscle group, but without utilizing weights.

12*a*. WEIGHT TRAINING WARM-UP

Purpose:	To utilize all of the major muscle groups in a warm-up routine prior to concentrating on specific muscle groups.
Starting Position:	Place feet astride; bend knees; keep back straight; hold a bar with an overhand grip (Position A).
Movement:	Straighten legs with back still straight; raise elbows to shoulder height or higher (Position B); lower elbows next to the trunk and keep the weight at chest level; press the weight over the head and fully extend arms (Position C); return weight to floor.
Repetitions:	8 to 10

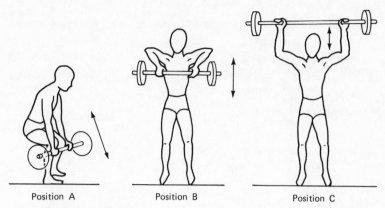

Position A Position B Position C

12b. JUMPING JACKS

Purpose: To utilize all of the major muscle groups in a warm-up routine prior to concentrating on specific muscle groups.

Starting Position: Stand erect with feet together and arms at the side.

Movement: Swing arms upward until over head and spread feet apart in one movement; in second movement, return to starting position.

Repetitions: 20

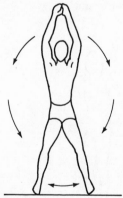

13. MILITARY PRESS

Purpose: To strengthen the shoulder, upper back, and arm muscles.

Starting Position: Support weight at shoulder level with an overhand grip.

Movement: Push weight directly overhead; keep the back and knees straight; return the weight slowly to starting position.

Repetitions: 10 to 12

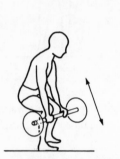 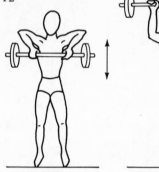 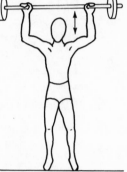

| Position A | Position B | Position C |

14*a*. CURL

Purpose: To strengthen the anterior arm muscles.

Starting Position: Hold weight with a palms-up grip; keep arms straight.

Movement: Bend arms and bring weight up to chest; return slowly.

Repetitions: 10 to 12

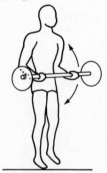

14*b*. PULL-UP

Purpose: To strengthen the anterior arm, upper back, and

shoulder muscles.

Starting Position: Place hands about 18 inches apart on overhead bar with either a palms-in or a palms-out grip; keep arms straight in order to support the body.

Movement: Pull body up so chin comes above the bar; slowly lower the body to starting position.

Repetitions: Progress to 10 to 15

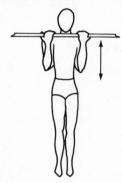

15*a*. SIT-UP

Purpose: To strengthen the abdominal and hip flexor muscles.

Starting Position: Lie on back with knees bent and hands clasped under head or holding weight on chest.

Movement: Raise head and trunk to an upright position; hold position for three counts; slowly return to starting position. Emphasize a roll-up type movement.

Repetitions: 15 to 20

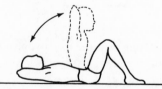

15*b*. LEG PULL-UP

Purpose: To strengthen the abdominal and hip flex or muscles.

Starting Position: Hang from bar with body straight.

Movement: Bend knees slowly; bring kness to chest; return slowly to starting position.

Repetitions: Progress to 10 to 15

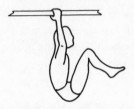

16a. BENT-OVER ROWING

Purpose: To strengthen the mid to upper back and posterior arm muscles.

Starting Position: Stand with feet apart slightly more than shoulder width; bend forward at waist with back straight and legs slightly bent; keep arms straight to support the weight.

Movement: Raise weight to chest and return it slowly to starting position.

Repetitions: 10 to 12

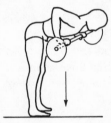

16b. PULL-UP, WIDE GRIP

Purpose: To strengthen the mid to upper back and the posterior and anterior arm muscles.

Starting Position: Place hands about 24 inches apart on overhead bar with either a palms-in or palms-out grip; hang from the bar with arms straight to support the body.

Movement: Pull body up so chin comes above the bar; slowly lower the body to starting position.

Repetitions: Progress to 10 to 15

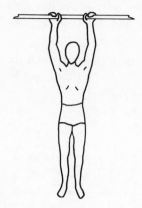

17a. SUPINE PRESS (BENCH PRESS)

Purpose:	To strengthen the chest, anterior shoulder, and posterior arm muscles.
Starting Position:	Lie on back on a bench 10 to 14 inches wide; use an overhand grip on a weight supported on standards or held by two assistants; keep arms straight.
Movement:	Slowly lower weight to touch the chest; raise weight until arms are straight.
Repetitions:	10 to 12

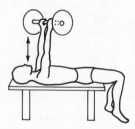

17b. PUSHUPS

Purpose:	To strengthen the chest, anterior shoulder, and posterior arm muscles.
Starting Position:	Lie on stomach with hands flat on floor and positioned beneath the shoulders.

Movement: Push entire body except feet and hands off the floor until the arms are straight; lower body until chest touches floor.

Note: Positioning the hands beyond the shoulders or putting blocks beneath the hands increases the stretch of the pectorals.

Repetitions: Progress to 20 to 30

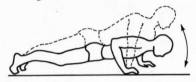

18*a*. BACK EXTENSION

Purpose: To strengthen the lower back muscles.

Starting Position: Lie on a bench with the face down; extend the body from above the waist over the edge of the bench; strap or hold the feet to the other end of the bench.

Movement: Lift head and trunk; slowly lower head and trunk.
Note: Do not hyperextend.
Repetitions: Progress to 10 to 15.

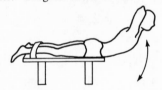

18*b*. BACK TIGHTENER

Purpose: To strengthen the lower back muscles.

Starting Position: Lie on floor with face down; fold hands over lower back area.

Movement: Raise head and chest and tense the gluteal and lower back muscles.

Caution: Do not hyperextend; just raise head and chest slightly off the floor; concentrate mainly on tensing gluteal muscles.

Repetitions: 10 to 15

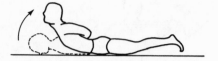

19. SQUAT

Purpose: To strengthen the anterior thigh and buttock muscles.

Starting Position: Stand erect with feet astride and support weight on shoulders with palms-up grip.

Movement: Keep the back straight and bend knees into a squat position; return to the standing position.

Note: Do half squat if knees are weak.

Repetitions: 10 to 12

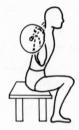

20a. HEEL RAISES (WITH WEIGHTS)

Purpose: To strengthen the calf muscles.

Starting Position: Place feet astride and hold weight on shoulders with a palms-up grip.

Movement: Raise to a toe position; lower body.

Note: A board may be placed under the toes to increase the range of motion.

Repetition: 10 to 15

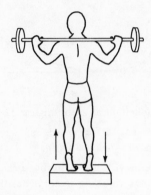

20*b*. HEEL RAISES

   Purpose: To strengthen the calf muscles.

Starting Position: Place feet astride and use arms for balance if necessary.

  Movement: Raise to a toe position; lower body.

    Note: A board may be placed under the toes to increase the range of motion.

  Repetition: 10 to 15

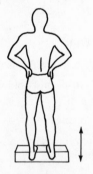

SUMMARY

General guidelines for exercise prescription are discussed. The exercise prescription is based upon the results from the participant's medical screening and fitness examination. We emphasize a specially individualized exercise prescription that is based on the participant's need, interest, and physical and health status. Special recommendations as to frequency, intensity, and duration of training are recommended for beginners and advanced exercisers. Individualized six-week starter programs and 20-week conditioning programs for walking and jogging are also outlined.

We stress that the total energy cost of the exercise program is the important factor in exercise prescription and emphasize that these calories can be expended through a variety of physical activities; thus participants should pick the activity(ies) that they enjoy. The notion that exercise should be done on a regular basis is emphasized.

Special exercises are described that can be used for developing and maintaining muscular strength and endurance, and flexibility. The exercises are categorized as to the specific area(s) of the body that they affect and are grouped in order of complexity. Both calisthenic exercises that need no special equipment and weight training exercises are listed.

Finally, certain hints as to precautions and proper exercise prescription for high-risk and cardiac patients are outlined.

REFERENCES

1. Balke, B. "Prescribing physical activity." In: *Sports Medicine*, L. Larson (ed). New York: Academic Press, 1974, pp 505-523.

2. Bruce, R.A. "Exercise testing of patients with coronary heart disease." *Ann. Clin. Res., 3*:323-332 (1971).

3. Cooper, K. *Aerobics.* New York: Bantam Books, 1968.

4. Cooper, K. *The New Aerobics.* New York: J.B. Lippincott, 1970.

5. Fox, S.M., J.P. Naughton, and W.L. Haskell. "Physical activity and the prevention of coronary heart disease." *Ann. Clin. Res., 3*:404-432 (1971).

6. *Guidelines for Graded Exercise Testing and Exercise Prescription.* Philadelphia,: Lea and Febiger, 1975.

7. Hooks, G. *Application of Weight Training to Athletics.* Englewood Cliffs, N.J.: Prentice-Hall, 1970.

8. Karvonen, M., K. Kentala, and O. Muslala. "The effects of training heart rate: a longitudinal study." *Ann. Med. Exptl. Biol. Fenn., 35*:307-315 (1957).

9. Kasch, F.W., and J.L. Boyer, *Adult Fitness Principles and Prac-*

tices. San Diego: San Diego State College, 1968.

10. Lind, A.R., D. Phil, and G. McNicol. "Muscular factors which determine the cardiovascular responses to sustained and rhythmic exercise." *Canad. Med. Ass. J., 96*:706-713 (1967).

11. Naughton, J.P., and H.K. Hellerstein (eds.). *Exercise Testing and Exercise Training in Coronary Heart Disease.* New York: Academic Press, 1973.

12. Pollock, M.L., J. Broida, and Z. Kendrick. "Validation of the palpation technique for estimation of training heart rate." *Res. Quart., 43*:77-81 (1972).

13. Pollock, M.L. "The quantification of endurance training programs." In: *Exercise and Sport Sciences Reviews,* Vol. 1 Wilmore, J. (ed.). New York: Academic Press, 1973, pp. 155-188.

14. Pollock, M.L. "Steps for initiating an endurance exercise program." *Rec. Manag., 17*:26-32 (1974).

15. Pollock, M.L., L.R. Gettman, C.A. Milesis, M.D. Bah, L. Durstine, and R.B. Johnson. "Effects of frequency and duration of training on attrition and incidence of injury. *Med. Sci. Sports, 9*: 31-36 (1977).

16. Rasch, P.J. *Weight Training.* Dubuque, Iowa: W.C. Brown, 1966.

17. Wilmore, J. "Individual exercise prescription." *Am. J. Cardiol., 33*: 757-759 (1974).

Section 5
Cardiac Rehabilitation

Cardiac rehabilitation can be considered the process of restoring spiritual, psychological, physical, and social functions to optimal levels. The role of *physical exercise* in enhancing each of these areas is of great significance. Although those of us who have worked with cardiac patients are impressed with the value of these activity programs, benefits are likely to extend far beyond this cardiovascular group. Undoubtedly, there is an even larger segment of the population whose physical and psychological health would benefit from the predictable boost associated with a program of rewarding physical activities.

Physical medicine and rehabilitation specialists have been recognized for the excellent results achieved with exercise after poliomyelitis, multiple fractures, trauma, musculoskeletal disorders, and diseases of the nervous system. Likewise, physical activity is frequently recommended after extensive breast, pelvic, and other cancer surgery when the lymphatic or venous drainage systems have been removed or compromised. In most areas, third party insurance carriers will provide such short-term programs with at least partial support.

In the field of rehabilitation for cardiac diseases, however, there has been much less financial support and, until recently, professional acceptance. The past 30 years have seen a profound shift away from the conservative approach that discouraged anginal and heart attack patients from becoming as active as their symptoms and hazard status might have permitted. Many were told to resign from the golf club and some to stop driving their cars and climbing stairs. Fortunately, Drs. Paul Dudley White, Samuel A. Levine, and Herman K. Hellerstein questioned this pessimistic and conservative approach. Respectively, they demonstrated the safety of activity for the anginal patient, the early use of a bedside chair for the stabilized heart attack victim, and progressive, endurance stimulating exercises for those whose infarcts had healed.

There is still difficulty, however, in obtaining health insurance support for cardiac rehabilitation. This is true both within the hospital and after discharge, when a significant change in life-style is more difficult to sustain. Part of this reluctance comes from the huge numbers of post infarct survivors—some 500,000 or more in the United States each year. Part may be due to the lack of the more visible signs of temporary disability—no cast, brace, surgical scars, or faltering step that will disappear or be less obvious after short-term rehabilitation. Finally, part of the reluctance stems from fears that because vigorous exercise may precipitate hazardous complications in a coronary patient, there would be no easily defined end point at which the rehabilitation program could be considered to have achieved an adequate effect.

Although deaths have occurred in such programs, they have been infrequent. Even life threatening dysrhythmias, particularly ventricular fibrillation, are rare. In one large, supervised program, all 17 such occurrences were corrected without evidence of new heart muscle damage (infarction). That program has reported one such ventricular fibrillation for an average of 6000 man-hours of vigorous gym activity. Others have had no such problems through over 100,000 man-hours. There appears to be a U.S. national average of one such life—threatening event for approximately 30,000 supervised program man hours. Therefore, it has been shown that properly supervised cardiac rehabilitation programs are reassuringly safe from life threatening events.

As yet, there are no long-term studies proving financial savings or benefits among those who had a program of cardiac rehabilitation as compared to those who had adequate acute care and were encouraged to change their life-style using their own mental, physical, and financial resources. Although there are ongoing studies in both the United States and Canada, the small number of subjects may lead to a "false negative" conclusion: the inability to demonstrate a significant benefit when a true difference could be shown if an adequate number of subjects were studied for a longer period of time. This is a very real hazard of doing well planned studies at an inadequate level of support.

An attempt at such a study was undertaken in Gothenburg (Göteborg) Sweden. After almost two years, it showed promise of demonstrating both significantly fewer deaths and a lesser reinfarction rate in those under physical training as compared to the randomly assigned control group (Table 5.1, Figures 5.1 and 5.2). Unfortunately, over half of the 111 people in the training group dropped out of active participation in the first year. Although randomized in the hospital, no evaluation or start of physical training occurred until three months postinfarction. Even then, there was a variable time with each patient before the physical training progressed to a level of probable significance. Thus, at least 13 and probably close to 17 or 20 weeks were included in the study before the physical activity levels were significantly different.

Until cardiac rehabilitation programs can be shown to diminish the recurrence rate or provide financial savings, it appears appropriate to justify the time, effort, and resources required on the basis of the physiological (physical function) and psychological benefits. The renewed sense of enthusiasm, optimism, and vigor that develop in the physically active individual will increase the quality in all aspects of his or her life.

Numerous cardiac rehabilitation services have been found useful. Table 5.2 presents some of the more frequently established programs.

It is important to indicate that few medical centers provide all the elements listed in a comprehensive cardiac rehabilitation program. Therefore, is would be unwarranted for a patient to feel neglected if the designated program or implied services were not provided during his or her convalescence. Also, it should be recognized that many patients do not need to progress through all the named stages in postinfarct rehabilitation—many can skip more rapidly to some more advanced phase. In all approaches, however, it is crucial to establish an understanding of the reasons behind a change in lifestyle.

Many professionals involved in cardiac rehabilitation find the educational aspects of the patient's participation to be even more critical than the physical activities themselves. An adequate understanding of atherosclerotic coronary and peripheral vascular disease involves awareness of its complex, multidimensional nature. Without such awareness,

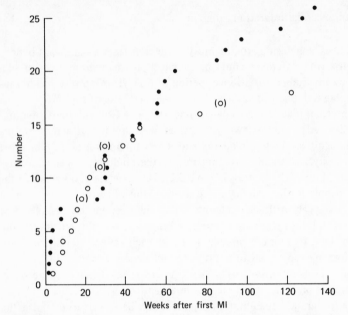

FIGURE 5.1. Accumulated number of deaths in the original groups randomized to training and to control in the Göteborg study of Sanne et al. It can be seen that there were fewer deaths in the training group (open circles) after 60 weeks than in the controls (filled circles). Brackets denote deaths due to other reasons than coronary heart disease. The follow-up beyond 140 weeks became less meaningful because of a high drop-out rate. (Courtesy of the authors and publisher.)

the patient is unlikely to undertake the following life-style changes that are necessary along with an exercise program:

1. Stopping smoking.
2. Reduction of body weight and serum lipids (fats) through modification of eating habits.
3. Adherence to the prescribed regimen of antihypertensive medication if medically indicated.

Less well established are the importance of controlling diabetes and the role of decreasing psychic "stress" and "strain". Exercise reduces the need for insulin for those diabetics requiring its use, although severe exercise can induce hazardously low blood sugar levels. Physical activity is also likely to help individuals deal with stress and strain, and reduce tension and anxiety. All in all, exercise may be the keystone of a total program of life-style revision.

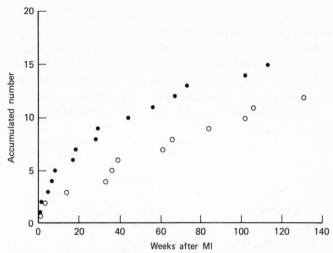

FIGURE 5.2. Accumulated number of reinfarctions in the original groups randomized to training and to control. It can be seen that the lesser occurrence of reinfarctions in the training group occurred early in the study but the trends were then parallel rather than continuing to diverge. Training group in open circles and control group in closed circles.

POSTMYOCARDIAL INFARCTION PROGRAM

IN HOSPITAL PHASE. Although there have been reports from Britain suggesting that some heart attack patients do as well at home as they do in the hospital, current U.S. and Canadian opinion is overwhelmingly to the contrary. The consensus is that hospitalization in a specifically organized unit with a specialized staff is appropriate for anyone suspected of having an acute coronary event. This includes patients with new or more extensive damage, as well as those with persistent chest discomfort not adequately explained by noncoronary factors. The significance of such discomfort should be determined by a careful review of symptoms and what influences them (arm movement, deep breathing, belching, etc), as well as physical and laboratory findings.

Once in a coronary care unit, or its equivalent, the first priorities are the avoidance of deterioration and the stabilization of adequate heart rhythm, pump function, blood pressure, ventilation of the lungs, and individual patient morale. The very fact that the patient has arrived in the unit indicates that he or she has survived the time and circum-

TABLE 5.1. Effect of physical training. Myocardial infarction patients, born 1913 and later, living in Göteborg, who became ill during the years 1968 to 1970. It can be seen that of 156 patients randomly assigned to training when in the coronary care unit, only 111 actually started training. It was only after the first 26 weeks of training that a statistically significant difference was found between the training and control groups relative to total deaths and those considered due to coronary heart disease.

Total number		316	
Randomized to	**TRAINING**		**CONTROL**
	156		160
Surviving 3 months	151		153
Started training	111		0
Mean follow up time (yr)	1.85		1.85
Mortality before Jun, 30, 71			
Total	18		26
Due to CHD	15		25
Mortality 26 weeks after MI and later:			
Total	8	$p < 0.05$	19
Due to CHD	6	$p < 0.025$	18

Reproduced with permission from H. Sanne, D. Elmfeldt, and L. Wilhelmsen. "Preventive effect of physical training after a myocardial infarction." In *Preventive Cardiology*, G. Tibblin, A. Keys and L. Werkö (eds.). Wiley, New York, 1972.

TABLE 5.2. Types of cardiac rehabilitation programs

I. POSTMYOCARDIAL INFARCTION PROGRAMS

    A. In hospital phase
    B. Continued healing phase
    C. Closely monitored phase
    D. Supervised group phase
    E. Independent phase

II. PRESURGICAL AND POSTSURGICAL PROGRAMS

    A. In hospital phase

B. Continued healing phase
C. Follow-on phase

III. ANGINA WITHOUT INFARCTION PROGRAMS

IV. PERIPHERAL VASCULAR PROGRAMS

V. PROGRAMS FOR OTHER CARDIOVASCULAR DISEASES

Arterial hypertension
Pulmonary hypertension
Assymetric Septal hypertrophy
Mitral prolapse
Heart block

VI. PREVENTIVE PROGRAMS FOR THOSE WITH HIGH RISK FACTOR STATUS

TABLE 5.3. Postmyocardial infarction rehabilitation program—in hospital.

LEVEL I—Initiated as soon as patient can comply and after physician clearance.
      Supine or with head of bed elevated for comfort.
      Three (3) "rounds" per day, preferably more.

1. Diaphragmatic (abdominal) breathing, 6 slow, deep breaths, avoid hyperventilation.
2. Active ankle plantar and dorsiflexion, 6 each, 3 times a day.
3. Partial passive range of motion (ROM) to all extremities, 4 each, 3 times a day, and performed slowly.

LEVEL II—Started as soon as a patient's clinical status permits (no hypotension, nor life-threatening dysrhythmia).
      Same position or as indicated-supervised.
      Four (4) "rounds" per day.

1. Repeat level I-perhaps increase to 4 times a day.
2. Full passive and progress to active ROM to all extremities, 4 times each, 4 times a day.
3. Head rotation—leading with the chin.
4. Sitting in chair, initially 10 minutes twice a day before meals, with support hose and with active ankle plantar and dorsiflexion.

5. Walking—only to commode and for sitting.
6. Start of education program including relaxation techniques—as physician wishes.

LEVEL III—Often appropriate on 5th to 7th day in uncomplicated cases.
Supine for No. 2, some of No. 1; all others sitting on edge of bed with feet supported or patient in chair.
Four (4) "rounds" per day.

1. Repeat Level II with supervised, unassisted active motion.
2. Alternate slow leg, hip, and knee flexion with feet in air (upside-down bicycling).
3. Shoulder trunk rotation—sitting with hands on bed.
4. Both arms raised horizontally to side with deep diaphragmatic breathing—sitting.
5. Full head circles slowly from back to side, front, other side, back and reverse.
6. Sitting-expand possibly to include meals.
7. Walking—slow "amble", (1 mile per hour) for 1 to 2 minutes supervised, taking heart rate and rhythm, in adjacent hall outside room.
8. Review and continue education/relaxation program.
9. Review dietary habits/preferences and nutritional objectives.

LEVEL IV—After 3 to 7 comfortable days at Level III.
Sitting or preferably standing for most activities.
Four (4) or more "rounds" per day.

1. Repeat Level III activities with coaching as needed.
2. Lateral trunk bending with arms at sides.
3. High stepping, knees to waist level, in place.
4. Walking—1½ to 2 mile per hour "saunter" for 2 to 5 minutes taking heart rate every 1 to 2 minutes for 10 or 15-second count (see section 4 for technique).
5. Stepping 8 to 12 ascents of 8 to 9-inch step in 1 minute—take heart rate immediately after.
6. Review and continue education/relaxation program.
7. Nutrition review and counselling.
8. Assessment of occupational needs and recreation goals as part of total life-style review.
9. Predischarge exercise tolerance evaluation, usually not to exceed 4

or 5 METS or heart rate of 120 beats/min.

stances in which over 50 percent of heart attack deaths occur. This statistic emphasizes the importance of getting the (suspected) patient into a protected environment: a mobile intensive care unit (originally called a "heartmobile"), a well staffed and well equipped emergency room, or the specially organized in hospital unit.

It cannot be overemphasized that persons with chest discomfort should avail themselves of these coronary care services. Improved techniques can now determine the significance of this discomfort within a few days or less, leading to an appropriate early release for patients found to be at a level of low risk for catastrophe. This will encourage the patient to seek shelter in a well equipped and staffed hospital with less apprehension that he or she will lose excessive time until decisions can be made. The hazards of trying to "tough it out" can be irreversible damage or death.

Once stabilized in the unit, the patient will be interested in knowing when he or she can perform certain self-care activities: sitting on a bedside commode rather than using a bedpan, brushing one's teeth, washing the genital area, and so on. Antidysrhythmic medications (which can often revert dangerous heart rhythms) and other recent advances have made it possible for some patients to slip over onto a bedside commode for bowel movements after 24 hours or less. The energy cost of such maneuvers may be less than what a discomforted patient may exert on a bedpan.

Physical rehabilitation maneuvers are now becoming widely accepted to start, even before washing and commode privileges are granted. To a great extent, this is due to the persuasive experience of Dr. Nanette Wenger of Atlanta. She established a 14-stage program that appears in somewhat altered form in Table 5.3.

The first purpose of the active ankle movements included in the protocol of Table 5.3 is to help push blood more rapidly through the leg veins and back to the heart. This decreases the chance of thrombophlebitis (clotting in the veins) and the hazardous breaking off of such clots that can be carried to the lungs as "pulmonary emboli." In addition, such activity permits the patient to get involved in working toward his or her future health. This represents prompt involvment of the patient as a member of the rehabilitation team as contrasted with being an object on which rehabilitation techniques are applied.

Diaphragmatic or "belly" breathing helps avoid atelectasis of the lower lobes of the lung near the diaphragm, i.e. the collapse of some air spaces of the lung that makes gas exchange impossible in the involved segments. A nurse or trained assistant should initially provide instruction in these maneuvers, and the attending physician should emphasize their importance. We have found some patients—most typically those who have seen military service—have great difficulty in belly breathing when lying on their back, since they are used to elevating the ribs and chest. The maneuver is often easier for these patients if they try it when lying on their side.

While repetitions every waking hour may appear burdensome, frequent personalized contact of an active sort is of definite value. In addition, avoidance of thrombophlebitis and inadequate lung action are of major significance in reducing the complications of any hospitalization. This is particulary true when discomfort or pain inhibit deep breathing and movement.

Likewise, Stage II has both a psychological and a physiological justification. Even at the gentlest level, the fact that these exercises are aimed at preserving muscle strength and joint mobility indicates the staff's optimistic conviction that there is an *active* future for the patient. Also, the "stiff neck and shoulder syndrome," once an altogether too frequent complication of heart attack hospitalization, has been almost completely prevented by these active maneuvers. The "shoulder/arm syndrome," of nagging discomfort, weakness, and poor control, was once considered to be due to reflex nerve dysfunction. It now appears to have resulted from simple lack of motion where chest and arm pain had made patients fearful of any unncecessary motion. Preservation of a good range of head rotation is important for driving and parking. The mention of these capabilities often provides a sense of purpose to activities that otherwise may appear trivial.

The modern coronary care unit, with bedside and central monitors and refined emergency therapy, has made it acceptable to undertake early but low energy hip and shoulder motion at least twice a day. The use of a chair, also of great psychological support, will help stimulate normal responses in the veins and other vessels in the legs and abdomen. In turn, this helps maintain their capacity to react promptly to the increased blood pressures caused by their being lower than the level of the heart. Although this may appear to be a small point, it was emphasized quite dramatically in the popular mind during the manned space program. Upon return to the gravitational environment of the earth, even the previously most fit young astronauts found themselves light headed and wobbly of gait on first resuming the upright position. More marked deconditioning can be expected with bedrest under conditions of discomfort and apprehension.

While the educational program cannot be detailed here, it should be emphasized that many patients want to learn about the coronary event that has happened to them, its causes and implications. Their questions often require more time than can be easily handled only by a physician on the time pressured rounds of an overloaded day. Most physicians now realize that a well prepared slide show and a booklet of simple diagrams are far more instructive than their sketchy drawings on the back of a prescription blank or a clinical record. While the physician should strongly recommend and reinforce the presentation of materials, a well informed staff can usually provide more complete coverage of the causes and the therapeutic approach to a heart attack. The team approach can provide the repeated reviews that will satisfy an apprehensive patient and family. Further details of educational materials are beyond the scope of this book but can be obtained from the local chapter of the American Heart Association or from hospital cardiac rehabilitation centers.

Stage III includes sitting on the edge of the bed with feet supported. Leg "dangling" is no longer permitted in most hospitals because the pressure of the mattress edge under the thighs tends to block venous blood return to the heart. This pressure promotes the same clotting tendency in static blood that the sitting up was intended to avoid. Therefore, a chair should be placed under the feet to lift the knees and thighs off the edge of the bed when the patient is sitting up. The early supervised walking may be with a long electrocardiographic cable, radiotelemetry, or staff surveillance without direct monitoring. The latter is least preferable, but with competent personnel can be undertaken with low risk. The walking is a very slow "ambling" around the unit (at 1 to 1.25 miles per hour) with the aim to gain balance, coordination, and psychic uplift rather than to stimulate the heart.

Stage IV activities round out the program prior to discharge and permit much more flexibility in substituting a wide choice of maneuvers. The intent, as before, is to preserve function and avoid complications rather than to build strength and endurance. The latter comes only after the heart has had the opportunity to heal thoroughly (approximately 8 to 12 weeks).

Noticeable in their absence, perhaps, are both sit-ups and pushups. Although they may have a place later, they are usually inappropriate until the heart is less irritable and more completely healed. It is important, however, to build up abdominal strength in order to provide belly wall support that can protect the back when lifting. Leg raises (knees bent) or upside down bicycling and the like can be used. High stepping is also good for abdominal and back development. The knees should be brought up as high as is comfortable but not pulled into the chest by the arms. Whatever the exercise, do not hold your breath!

Repetitive stepping up and down using an 8- to 9-inch step can be done in a patient's room with small portable steps like those described in Appendix A, under step test. Rather than making the classic Master's trips over and down, the patient uses alternate feet up and back down one or two steps depending on clinical evaluation. A good time to test the pulse taking skill of the patient is after this stepping.

Many hospitals are now developing in patient cardiac rehabilitation centers. These in patient centers are equipped with treadmills, stationary bicycles, step benches and monitoring devices (radiotelemetry). In this way, the patient can be continuously monitored for dangerous symptoms while accomplishing a variety of tasks. The center provides for a more systematic and precise means of monitoring physical activity. The postinfarct patient will normally not report to the in patient center until after the 10th day and/or when stable.

It may be of considerable significance to know the patient's exercise tolerance prior to discharge from the hospital. The patient who has suffered a myocardial infarction or sudden catastrophic rhythm disturbance starts an exercise program with a more complex set of circumstances than the average hospitalized person. Various indices developed to characterize short- and long-term risk have been helpful in some aspects of patient management. The actual testing of the exercise response, however, is still the most relevant means for "clearance" for physical activities or for developing an exercise prescription.

At the annual meeting of the American College of Sports Medicine in 1973, Dr. Patrick A. Gorman reported on the first systematic assessment of treadmill evaluations prior to discharge from the usual three-week hospitalization for uncomplicated myocardial infarction. Electrocardiographic monitoring at low work intensity is important as an indicator of susceptibility to both rhythm disturbances and remaining areas of ischemia (inadequate blood supply to the heart). The intent is not to determine a maximum capacity, but to assure the patient and spouse that some options for minimal activity are feasible. It appears wise to limit the demands of the treadmill program to no more than 4 or 5 METS or 120 beats/min. usually achieved by walking no faster than 2 miles per hour at an incline 7 or 10.5 percent, respectively.

Not all infarct patients are considered ready for this type of evaluation before discharge. Some have severe or persistent disturbances of rhythm or poor circulatory capacity suggesting the need to limit activities to the absolute minimum. For those at a level where slow stair climbing and walking seems possible, however, it is reassuring to find there is little reason to restrict such activity in about two-thirds of the tested subjects. For the one-third who show less adequate responses, a repeat evaluation in three weeks is often helpful. For these patients, sexual activity and other elective energetic activities may not be advisable in the interim. Walking at a slow pace to avoid vein clotting and ankle swelling is recommended for the patient who can get about. Therefore, the individual is encouraged that he or she is making definite progress, even if deliberately slow.

One of the chief objectives of the predischarge exercise evaluation is to assess the risks of resuming sexual activity and to help compose a convincing presentation of the facts to both the patient and partner. Studies show that sexual intercourse with one's wife approximates a 5 MET level of work and in most cases is associated with a heart rate lower than 130 beats/min. Extra marital sex relations are likely to cause a higher heart rate response. Many physicians feel that if a patient can climb two flights of stairs at a moderate rate without complications (heart rate above 120 beats/min), then they are ready to resume sexual relations. For a psychologically hard-hit male struggling with strong depressive tendencies in the strange surroundings of a hospital, sex may be valued both for relief of tension and as a reassurance of future capability. The heart health team must instruct such a patient on how to achieve a healthy sex life through modifying the intensity and orchestrating the encounter with a light touch of low energy demand. It is especially important that the patient's partner have an explanation of the permission for low demand sexual activity to relieve the natural anxiety and fear of further heart damage. If the evaluation suggests that sex can be undertaken at acceptably low hazard, the postinfarct patient needs to be reassurred that he or she can enjoy sex and be an adequate partner. It is crucial to provide counsel in this area, although not easy, even with the help of an early discharge evaluation. It is also important that the physician or other designated members of the team initiate a discussion and solicit questions of partners in this area of continuing occasional embarrassment.

One of the major goals in an early postinfarct activity program is to provide psychological support while the damaged heart muscle is replaced with a strong scar that has been permitted to contract down to minimal size. Current opinion supports the findings of Drs. Kenneth Mallory, Paul Dudley White, and colleagues who demonstrated almost 40 years ago that it takes about three months for the scar to achieve relatively complete and strong repair. During that time, increases in either psychological or physical stress will tend to add stretching tension on the fibrous tissue forming the scar. Hence, activity privileges, however valuable for psychological and physical function (to avoid thromboembolism and loss of bone and muscle strength) must be balanced against damage to the still healing heart. Current philosphy in the rehabilitation of the postinfarct patient calls for low level maintenance activity for the first 8 to 12 weeks. After this healing period, developmental activities can then begin.

Psychologists, cardiologists, and coronary care nurses agree that patients are almost always threatened or engulfed in a significant and understandable depression at some time during convalescence from an infarct. Although medication is often indicated, the staff's demonstrated commitment to and expectation of the patient's restoration to a high quality of life is often most critical. This extends far beyond their responsibilities for patient survival. Education, evaluation, and training aimed at meaningful postdischarge activities demonstrate the team's optimism for a return to a life that can be even more satisfying than the time and responsibility pressured circumstances that often precede an infarct.

Upon discharge from the hospital, it is helpful to provide a schedule of anticipated activity that can be permitted (Tables 5.4 and 5.5). Activities such as starting and pushing a lawn mower should be deferred until much later, particularly if the weather is very hot or the terrain hilly. For estimated MET levels for exercise and leisure time activities, see Tables 4.3 and 4.4. Other items, such as when a patient can be left at home alone, depend on psychological status and clinical judgement of hazard.

THE CONTINUED HEALING PHASE. As mentioned earlier, the healing process continues for approximately three months, while tough fibrous tissue replaces the heart muscle lost to useful function during the acute episode. This fibrous scar needs much less nutritional blood supply than muscle to heal firmly and to contract down to a smaller than initial size—an important attribute of scar tissue. Vigorous exercise tends to stretch that tissue and thwart useful contraction.

After a week at home, the patient should return for an office visit to discuss modification of the home program. This is particulary important in terms of sexual activity, stair climbing, walking, and social contacts. During the first weeks after hospital discharge the main thrust is psychological support, avoidance of further bone and muscle deterioration, clotted veins, and urinary and bowel disfunction. Several visits a week to an outpatient exercise and education facility may add hope, optimism, and gentle activity. These benefits far outweigh the minimal hazard, expense, and inconvenience. Use of such devices as a stationary bicycle, rowing machine, small treadmill, shoulder-arm flexibility wheel, steps and arm resistance ergometer are recommended at very low intensities, particularly when emphasis on arms and legs is alternated as in the sequence described. This provides an opportunity for review of other home exercises including flexibility stretches, and the nutritional and medication programs. A suggested upper limit heart rate for such activity would approximate 120 beats/ min or 20 beats/min above standing rest.

THE CLOSELY MONITORED OUTPATIENT PHASE. After settling down to a regular routine at home, there tends to be another slide into discouragement, if not frank depression. A regular schedule of visits to a closely monitored rehabilitation program provides psychological benefits and increases the patient's ability to expand the range and intensity of activity. Through a formal circuit training approach with specific stations for certain activities, the individual feels a sense of accomplishment yet does not rush to the next activity without a rest break or a brief walk. These activities must be undertaken at a slow pace, starting with almost no resistance. Stretching and flexibility maneuvers are also of value. The use of electrocardiographic monitoring, either by "hard wire" connections to an oscilloscope and recorder, or by radiotelemetry, helps adjust the intensity and duration to appropriate levels. This support appears to be well worth the effort and necessary charges for at least one to two months, or until a 6 MET work load is sustained for three or more minutes without evidence of undue hazard or circulatory dysfunction. Costs can be reduced if four to eight patients proceed around the circuit of devices in close succession so that personnel and space expenses can be shared.

Participation in a structured rehabilitation program also provides the opportunity to expand on the previous educational program. Often, it is necessary to repeat much of the information provided while the patient was in the hospital. Initial apprehension may impede retention of information soon after the patient's infarct, yet the very fact that the staff refers to a time beyond mere "survival" gives as much reassurance as many direct statements of good progress. Likewise, the almost inevitable postinfarct depression makes retention and integration of facts difficult not only in the latter stages of hospitalization but also upon return home. The patient has to adjust to at least temporary loss of his or her previous position of authority.

SUPERVISED GROUP PHASE. Upon achieving a 6 MET capacity, most patients can transfer from the continuously monitored program to one in which 20 or more patients are taking part in a supervised program of stretching and muscle conditioning, and endurance activities. Initially, a new patient may perform a limited number of the repetitions of each exercise, perhaps 4 or 6 out of a total of 12, and then rest. Or the patients may do one repetition and skip one or two so that six or four, respectively, slow repetitions are completed while others are doing 12. Likewise, he or she may walk three laps around a gym (20+ laps to a mile), jog down one side (10 to 15 paces), walk two or three sides and repeat. A large wall clock with a highly visible sweep second hand can be used for pacing and counting the pulse. This type program has become an important part of YMCA's, Jewish Community Centers, and some universities and colleges.

A question now asked is how long health insurance programs should supply funding for patient participation. When does rehabilitation end and continuing therapy begin? When a patient returns to work at a sedentary job, does this mean that health is sufficiently restored? We believe that a supervised program for a minimum of the first six months after an uncomplicated infarct is usually needed to provide adaquate rehabilitation to the patient. This period of time appears to be necessary to motivate the patient to continue the physical activities and make them

TABLE 5.4. Georgetown University Hospital posthospital discharge activities schedule

AROUND THE HOUSE	WEEK OF	WEEK OF	WEEK OF	WEEK OF
Up, dressed, about				
Back for bed rest				
Naps after meals				
Fix own hair				
Walk inside house				
Climb one flight				
Walk—your land				
Walk round block				
Sit in yard				
Sexual relations				
Beer, wine, cocktails				
Friends to visit				
Be left alone				
Help make bed				
Help cook/clean up				
Put out trash				
Pull weeds, water lawn				
Dust, vacuum				

TABLE 5.5. Georgetown University Hospital posthospital discharge activities schedule

OUTSIDE THE HOME	WEEK OF	WEEK OF	WEEK OF	WEEK OF	WEEK OF
Be driven in car					
Near walks alone					
Walk dog alone					
Attend religious services					
Attend nearby movie/play					
Visit friends					
Shopping—no carrying					
Grocery shopping					
Restaurant dinner					
Exercise tolerance evaluation					
Drive locally					
Work three hours					
Work two-thirds time					
Work full-time					
Drive to work					
Overnight trips					
Commercial air trips					
Three-day, longer trips					
Change auto tire					
Attend ball game					
Swim on back					
Swim arms in water					
Golf, with cart					

a regular part of a new life-style. For those with hazardous rhythm disturbances or other evidence of poor exertional response, an even longer period may be necessary.

As the patient returns to work, both the frequency of visits and the third party payments may have to be reduced. Patients may engage in more low intensity activities on their own time, although they may walk, swim, or participate in low intensity, low competition games (ping pong, social badminton, tennis doubles, volleyball) at the same facility. The movement toward more exercise programs for cardiac patients imposes requirements for professional competence, equipment, and training.

The fact that men who have been exercising regularly without incident for up to four years after a heart attack still get into potentially lethal problems suggests to some physicians and program directors that supervised programs are needed for almost every postinfarct patient—forever. Others cite low mortality figures and contend that with adequate precautions about intensity, emotions, cold, heat, and humidity, many patients can exercise on their own with acceptable low hazard. Some patients try to convince their physician that they can return to the squash or handball court. Our experience appears too meager, however, to state what criteria should be applied for such clearance. The fact that numerous postinfarct patients are running marathons clearly demonstrates the potential for outstanding results.

INDEPENDENT PHASE OF POSTINFARCT REHABILITATION. This phase is the most important in the patient's long term rehabilitation. The activities included should be rewarding, and preferably fun for the patient. Costs in time, facilities, and money should be within the patient's capability. A swimming, home exercise bicycle or walk-jog-run program can serve as the main activity.

Patients frequently need help in becoming comfortable joggers. Using the treadmill helps demonstrate the importance of placing the heel down first and then rolling forward gently until a soft push-up from the ball of the foot naturally occurs, with minimal vertical bounce. Many formerly athletic men, including past basketball and tennis players, can *run* but do not understand how to slow down to a low intensity jog. After a 10-minute fast walking warm-up, a 20 to 60 minute endurance phase begins, followed by a tapering off walk. To determine proper pace for the endurance phase of the program, check Section 4 for starter programs on other levels of conditioning. When and if the postinfarct patient is ready to shift from a walking program to a walk-jog routine, intermittent progression steps are needed prior to beginning the walk-jog starter program listed in Table 4.7. Initially, 110 yd jog segments maybe too demanding. Preferably begin the walk-jog sequence level shown in Table 4.7. From then on, the normal progression shown in Section 4 may be followed.

The use of the treadmill for demonstration may seem unnecessary and expensive, but the ability to hold the speed constant makes it easier to demonstrate and emphasize the slow speed indicated at the start. Some people also benefit from holding onto the handrails while they learn to plant their heels. Depending on leg length, previous activity, and mental approach, a speed of $3\frac{1}{2}$ to 4 miles per hour is sufficient until a person develops a smooth technique. As indicated in Section 7, it is important to insist on good "training shoes," which have far more heel protection than the lighter "running shoes" of competition. The thick athletic sock will not convert old sneakers into adequate footwear for jogging.

It is particularly important to emphasize the flexibility exercises that stretch the various muscle groups of the body. See Section 4 for recommendation for an exercise routine. Patients should initially avoid doing pushups or any other activity that causes breath holding.

For many patients, a swimming routine is optimal. More pool coordinators are reserving time and lanes for serious swimmers and welcome postcoronary patients. Cardiac rescusitation in a pool area, however, has added complexities. Special care should be taken by management to provide training for their personnel. Furthermore, the staff should be informed of the coronary patient's status.

If a patient cannot find a supervised group program, certain basic principles should be emphasized while exercising on his or her own. Increasing the frequency and duration of activity is preferable and less hazardous than a concentration on increased intensity.

Although golf is not a good stimulus to high level performance, it may help the postcoronary patient get back into a social schedule along with healthful activity. However, some people cannot play golf without considerable psychic tension, or they feel they are expected to put an "edge" on each hole with a bet. Frank discussions of these aspects are necessary. Some patients are better off not going back to golf until they develop a more relaxed approach. Unless the course is extremely hilly, it is usually better for the coronary golfer to walk rather than ride a cart. Some courses, however, require cart rental to make more money or to move people more rapidly between strokes. Such policies appear grossly counterproductive to the health enhancement of our citizens.

In time, the postcoronary patient may become more physically capable than prior to the infarct. It is not infrequent for patients to say they are almost glad they had the infarct, because it forced them to break out of a stressful and unfulfilling pattern and rebuild their activities into a more satisfying new life.

Exercise tolerance tests at 2 to 3, 6 and 9 or 12 months postinfarct are of considerable help in adjusting the exercise prescription and in supporting patient motivation. After the nine or 12 month exam (following six months of real training activity), the spacing of subsequent tests is a matter of clinical judgement and can be related to the intensity and interests of the subject. An evaluation before a hunting, skiing, or other strenuous trip would appear prudent, even if within six uncomplicated months of a previous exercise test demonstrating good reserves. Otherwise, an annual comprehensive evaluation and review of risk factors may serve the busy, intelligent patient whose compliance to all aspects of the program is good.

Many coronary patients are understandably concerned about their sexual performance. Until Hellerstein and Friedman studied the heart rate response of postinfarct males during marital relations, there was little understanding of the cardiac demands of these circumstances. They found that the peak heart rates during intercourse ranged from 101 to 121 beats per minute; the mean peak rate was 117. Two-thirds of those men who undertook physical training reported fewer symptoms during sexual intercourse as compared to before training.

Recently Dr. Richard Stein reported that with an 11½ percent increase in maximum oxygen transport capacity, his group of post infarct men had a reduction in peak coital heart rate from an average of 127 to 120 beats per minute after a 16-week bicycle ergometer training program, three times a week for 40 minutes. Physical training, therefore, has been found to enhance the capacity to undertake sexual activity and thus increases the margin of safety. In addition, it restores confidence and enthusiasm for all aspects of living.

We should caution our patients that the above mentioned studies related to intercourse with long time marital partners. The "Couplets"

of Dr. David Kritchevsky of the Wistar Institute in Philadelphia express
these concerns appropriately:

Couplets on Coronary Coupling

> Coronary, have a care
> Think before that new affair
> Dr. Zohman studied swingers
> And her facts are really zingers
>
> Sex domestic, also straight
> Hardly makes you palpitate
> Heart beats stay at normal rate
> When one beds with legal mate
> And the danger that it bears
> Looms like—well, two sets of stairs
>
> But roosting in another's nest
> Flirts with cardiac arrest
> End result of evening's sport is
> Very often rigor mortis
> So seduction's needs are three
> Soft lights, music, E K G.

More recently, a cardiovascular surgeon added these thoughts:

> But if it's essential to indulge your lust
> In the surgeon you can trust
> To your ischemic heart he'll bring
> The blood that's needed when you swing
>
> You Don Juans need not despair
> Go ahead—have your affair
> But keep in mind you risk your life
> There's no surgical cure for the angry wife.

PRESURGICAL AND POSTSURGICAL PROGRAMS

The cardiac patient is especially in need of optimal physical conditioning before any surgery. Postoperative progress may be greatly

influenced by good lung function, the ability to cough and clear the airways, and responsiveness of the peripheral vascular system. It is particularly valuable to have the good stroke volume (amount of blood pumped by the heart each beat) in the heart itself that comes from endurance stimulating preoperative physical activities. For these reasons, physicians believe it highly worthwhile to place a person on a preparatory program prior to any major heart surgery. After a myocardial infarction, it is of particular value to get a few months of preparation if circumstances permit. Sometimes, a patient's status requires rather precipitous surgery. The attempts at fat reduction and physical training have to give way to the urgent need.

A near starvation type of weight-reduction program is foolhardy, since it is almost unavoidable to lose protein stores and useful muscle as well as fat tissue. The obese patient, however, is predisposed at a significantly increased level to thrombophlebitis, embolism, pulmonary congestion, and atelectasis (collapse of the small air cells blocking effective gas exchange).

Some of the best preparatory exercises include trunk rotation (Section 4, No. 1), abdominal churn (No. 3b), the inverted stretch (No. 6), the advanced front leg stretch (No. 7c), side stretch (No. 8), situps (No. 15a), pullups (No. 14b), and a few push-ups (No. 17b), if the patient can tolerate them. In the immediate preoperative days, it is also worthwhile to instruct the patient relative to the maneuvers to be followed after recovery from anesthesia. Although the same routines used in the postinfarct patient have value, incisional discomfort may be a limiting factor. Other special exercises to be used by the pre and post surgical patient includes the following stretching exercises:

1. Using cane or long stick; arms down in front; lift straight over head, down behind head, straight over head again, then down in front. Count to 4, 10 to 15 repetitions.
2. Using cane or long stick; put cane behind back of neck, push up as far as possible. 10 to 15 repetitions.
3. Using cane or long stick; put cane behind lower back, lift up and down. 10 to 15 repetitions.
4. Using cane or long stick; arms and hands in front of body, swing arms from side to side up to shoulder level. 10 to 15 repetitions.
5. Spinal twist; swing arms and twist body from side to side. 10 repetitions in each direction.

6. Lateral flexion; swing arm up high over head as trunk bends to opposite side. 10 repetitions in each direction.

7. Chicken wings; hands on top of shoulders elbows out, rotate forward and backward. 10 to 15 repetitions in each direction.

IN HOSPITAL POSTSURGICAL PHASE. Since the patient in the immediate postoperative phase will be partially sedated and confused, prior instruction in diaphragmatic "belly" breathing will prove to be highly worthwhile. Coughing will be painful for some, but having a person apply side pressure on the chest while such attempts are made may be helpful. This is a better practice then the old round-the-chest bandages that inhibited good breathing and coughing efforts. Along with the clinical and surgical assessment of the patient's capability, the nature of the incision and the type operation will influence the program. Sitting in a chair and walking may be limited because of intravenous infusion units and other attached apparatus. However, sitting on the side of the bed with feet warm and supported by a chair (and with thromboembolism deterring stockings) should often be accomplished the first day postoperation. Also, slow ambulation around ward is very common during the second day.

A major consideration with chest surgery (thoracotomy, or opening the chest) is the discomfort with many movements, yet the urgency to clear the airways to permit good lung function and avoid complications. Fortunately few patients recall more than a hazy period of discomfort for a few days and thus should not be fearful of recurrent bad dreams of pain and suffering.

Although the bowel is cleared out preoperatively, it is often uncomfortable for the patient to strain at stool when the need arises—usually two or three days after surgery. Good abdominal muscle tone and the ability to get to a bedside commode can both be helped by preoperative exercises. Assistance in movement is helpful and at times absolutely necessary to avoid sudden muscle pulls and the painful discouragement that can result. Fluid and electrolyte balances may be more disturbed than after an uncomplicated infarct and thus predispose the patient to postural blood pressure changes and light headedness for approximately one week postoperatively.

It is important to start both shoulder and neck mobility exercises as soon as they are tolerated (see stretching exercises listed above). Usually, these involve passive motion with a nurse or therapist moving the arms and the patient rolling the head gently from side to side.

With early assistance, such as elbow support, the patient can brush his or her own teeth and use an electric razor. Fixing the hair is more demanding and can initially be done by an attendant, relative, or friend. Washing the anterior genital area can be done without much distress but wiping and washing posteriorly—even on a bedside commode—requires more incisional and muscle pull. Initially this may best be done by others. This degree of detail is provided to help patients recognize that such activities are to be expected and that the staff is fully prepared to support the patient by providing all necessary services. It is also encouraging that those who are more fit preoperatively are more promptly able to resume self-care activities.

As discomfort subsides and the staff permits more activity, the patient will be assisted in walking and in efforts to regain a fully upright posture. In this area, the emphasis is greater than with the postinfarct patient.

The exercise rehabilitation program can generally progress more rapidly for the surgical patient. The uncomplicated postsurgical patients can begin to progress and increase their workload as soon as they feel up to it. The endurance exercise is still of low intensity but the duration can be increased at a faster rate than the infarction patient. Other aspects of the inhospital program are similar as described for infarct patients, that is, patient education, etc. The target heart rate can be up to 130 beats/min or 30 beats/min above standing rest for the uncomplicated surgical patient. Also, once the patient is free from various tubes and monitoring devices, walks should be taken three to four times daily.

Discharge from the hospital may be as soon as within the week. For heart valve replacement patients, however, discharge may be deferred considerably. The mechanical valves require lifetime anticoagulant therapy, while valves from other animals may require only a preliminary period.

The coronary bypass patient may have had the saphenous vein removed from one or both legs. Hence, he or she can expect local soreness and swelling resulting from the need to open up other veins to take the flow. Exercise helps reduce some of this swelling, if done with adequate support hose. It may take weeks, however, to get the leg totally comfortable and back to normal size. It will also be discolored with a variety of colors until the inevitably leaked blood pigments are slowly removed from the leg.

For the golfer, tennis player, and other sport enthusiasts, it is particularly important to start a flexibility program as soon as possible. Much of this will be initiated or continued out of the hospital.

THE CONTINUED HEALING PHASE. As with the postinfarct patient, it is important to provide a good program for home use after discharge. Initially this will be of the low-energy type to permit strong healing of grafts, incisions through the heart muscle, or sites of placement of artificial valves or repair patches. Depending on the nature and complications of the surgery, the patient can return relatively rapidly to activities that do not put stress on incisions and suture lines. In the past, 15 percent or more of coronary bypass operations had some myocardial infarction occurring along with the beneficial bypass. Better techniques are reducing this complication, but it is difficult to know if, and how much, such damage might have occurred. Light arm exercises are therefore preferable to pushups, heavy lifting, or strenous activities like snow shovelling, or turning over the compost pile. We caution the patient who can drive a car to call for assistance if he or she has a flat tire. Later in the convalescence, the patient can take a break between each short effort in the procedure. Changing a tire can be done with low-energy demands but the patient must be sure to rest frequently.

If the postbypass patient is uncomplicated, then he or she may begin with one of the starter programs listed in Section 4. Generally just the walking program would be recommended in the early continued healing phase. Depending on the patient's 8 to 12 week exercise tolerence test results, the responsible physician may then recommend jogging or other higher intensity activities. The latter activities should progress slowly.

THE FOLLOW-ON PHASE. We all wish that surgery would totally correct the problems that indicated its use; some heart problems can be totally corrected by surgery but many cannot. In regard to coronary surgery, however, the process of atherosclerosis will still proceed unless all risk factors are given optimal attention. In some areas, we don't know exactly what "optimal" is. We do know, however, how to deal with smoking and obesity—eliminate both, with smoking the most important. Good blood pressure control is clearly prudent and of proven benefit relative to some noncoronary complications as indicated in Section I. Dietary control of cholesterol, triglycerides and low-density lipoproteins is also highly recommended. Good dietary and, where necessary, insulin control of diabetes is considered important. Reordering priorities and schedules to reduce psychic stress and strain is not easy. However, this may be one of the most important changes that will enhance the quality of life, whatever its length may be.

For the postoperative patient as well as the individual recovering from an infarct, it is not known exactly how much exercise should be included. It can be argued that the fibrinolysis stimulating action of exercise has particular relevance to a postcoronary bypass patient, although we know of no data supporting this apparently logical view.

While the patient may have major relief of symptoms and hopefully hazardous ischemic areas, it is essential that he or she understand that the basic disease is still likely to continue despite many prudent life-style changes.

ANGINA PECTORIS PROGRAMS

Angina pectoris is the "squeeze or strangling in the breast" (chest by modern usage) first and best described by William Heberden in 1772. Although actual pain is present in moderately severe cases, angina is more frequently experienced as a severe discomfort or sense of constriction behind the breast bone. Radiation of the discomfort up to the neck, jaw, individual teeth, or arms is a typical occurence. Since the appearance of anginal symptoms can be quite varied, upper abdominal discomfort without the chest component must be taken seriously. In most cases, the discomfort is induced by physical exertion, sometimes by astonishingly low levels of activity such as combing one's hair or other arm elevation maneuvers. It is also of interest that Heberden described a woodcutter who had to stop his work in the early-morning stages because of angina, yet later in the day could engage in more vigorous and intense activity with little or no symptoms. We have had to rediscover this "warm-up" phenomenon in recent years among exercising patients.

The symptoms of angina can provide a warning to the individual approximately proportional to the electrocardiographic evidence of inadequate blood supply to the heart muscle. Thus, the discomfort can be interpreted as a signal to ease back on either exertional intensity or psychological involvement. There are many persons, however, who do not develop such discomfort even with a well documented myocardial infarction. Where no reliable discomfort occurs, the physician and heart health team must provide other means of avoiding overexertion, such as the heart rate response or detection of pulse irregularities. When the patient does recognize chest discomfort, it can be a useful guide to setting the appropriate adjustments for such influences as cold, heat, humidity, previous meals, or a continued psychological burden after a tense situation.

Because the perception of pain differs widely, attempts to grade the degree of discomfort on some simple scale have been extremely difficult. A rating from Grade 1 to 4 has been useful, although more precise assessment would be preferable.

Grade 1 is the discomfort that is established—but just established. Some patients speak of Grade ½ discomfort as that premonitory sensation that precedes the Grade 1 level as they walk, have sex, or get emotionally upset.

Grade 2 discomfort is that from which one can be distracted by a noncataclysmic event. It can be "pain," but usually is not.

Grade 3 discomfort or pain prevents distraction by a pretty girl, handsome man, a TV show or other consuming interest. Only a tornado, earthquake, or explosion, can distract one from grade 3 discomfort or pain. During exercise testing, it should rarely be permitted for long, even when no other evidence of danger exists. In an unsupervised situation, it should definitely be avoided.

Grade 4, or maximal discomfort or pain, is the most excruciating experienced or imaginable. It should be avoided completely.

Grade 3 anginal discomfort is often relieved or at least eased by a sublingual tablet of nitroglycerin, which lessens the work of the heart by reducing peripheral resistance. Before climbing a hill, starting the lawn mower, or sexual intercourse, some form of nitroglycerine preparation may also be of prophylactic use to avoid or lessen anginal pain.

The anginal patient should carry a small, tightly stoppered dark brown bottle of nitroglycerin tablets and insure their freshness by replacing them at least every six months. Storage in the refrigerator when at home may help preserve effectiveness. The nitroglycerin is sufficiently strong if it has a sharp, bitey taste and gives a pounding in the head if not a brief (10 to 20 minute) headache.

The effective action of nitroglycerin should occur in one to three minutes and last 10 to 30 minutes. If relief does not occur, one or two repeat tablets can be taken at five-minute intervals. Pain for more than 15 minutes that persists after three rounds of active nitroglycerin tablets is usually considered sufficient cause to be taken to a hospital emergency room or similar facility.

Other forms of nitroglycerin or related compounds include a paste that is applied to a strip of flexible plastic and taped to the arm, chest, or abdomen. In some cases, the long action resulting from slow absorption through the skin gives superior relief. Frequently, this method is useful even for activities where considerable sweating occurs.

Many patients do particularly well with a long acting nitrate and a Beta-blocking agent. Although the microscopic structure of the Beta transmission site in nerve tissue has not been identified, the concept of a "junction box" is useful in describing the transmission of sympathetic stimulation of the "fight or flight" reaction. This reaction almost routinely gives the healthy heart a faster rate, a more vigorous contraction, and a higher blood pressure at the start of exercise. Although these reactions were helpful in less civilized times, they may be more demanding than we need to maintain a moderate, long-term useful effort. In proper dosage, a good Beta blocker permits more total body work with less heart muscle oxygen and blood supply requirements— a pharmacological resetting of efficiency. The end result is a lower heart rate for a standard work load.

In the United States at present, only the Beta blocker, propanolol, is generally available. Other agents, however, are being used successfully in Europe and may soon be approved by the Food and Drug Administration.

Unfortunately, Propanolol, along with all its virtues, has an occasional tendency to reduce the vigor of heart action to an undesirable level. In addition, this medication may aggravate airway obstructions of the asthmatic type. In these cases, reevaluation or readjustment of the prescription may be necessary. This is primarily the responsibility of physicians, but physical educators, nurses, and other knowledgeable members of the team can help the patient become a skillfull adjuster of dose and timing of antianginal drugs. This will permit a wider range of activities with little, if any, increase in hazard. These agents do not appear to decrease the sensitivity to anginal discomfort but rather reduce the work of the heart involved in the total body activity.

Patients often find that angina of effort is actually helpful in gauging the safe limits of activity. Some concern may be appropriate when the angina patient goes swimming. From anecdotal reports, there is suggestion that swimming decreases the awareness of angina symptoms. This may be due to the competitive sensation of water contact to the chest, neck, face, and so on. Some individuals have a slowing of the heart when their face or other skin areas are in the water—similar to the intriguing "diving reflex" of seals.

In some cases, heart patients may enjoy a low-level cooling walk in the water when they are not yet ready to actively use their arms to swim. Recent data suggest that walking chest deep in water will often be associated with a lower pulse for a given total body oxygen consumption than if a person is on dry land.

It is important to realize that the anginal patient can often get good and seemingly safe relief from discomfort through an exercise program. Through careful pacing of his or her efforts and the support of some very effective drugs, a wider range of activity can be realized. We must work with anginal patients to instruct them in these techniques and encourage them to try different activities and approaches. The improvement in exercise tolerance in anginal patients who conscientiously work at a good program is convincing proof of the benefits exercise can provide the heart.

PERIPHERAL VASCULAR DISEASE

This term refers to disorders of the circulation occurring at a distance from the heart. (The cerebrovascular system is considered distinct and is controlled by separate factors).

With exercise training, important and subtle changes occur in the circulation to the abdominal organs (the mesenteric circulation) and to the kidneys. At rest the kidneys use approximately 25 percent of total cardiac output but can get along with very little during an hour of exercise. With a regular and progressively more vigorous activity program, more appropriate constriction of arterial blood supply to the intestines and kidneys is likely to develop. This permits more total body activity at lesser power requirements for the heart.

The same economy of circulatory distribution applies to the hiker, bicycler, and runner who doesn't need much blood to the arms but desires maximal circulation to the legs at the lowest level of demand on the heart. The well conditioned athlete will regulate the flow of blood to all areas in a manner that satisfies specific needs without permitting excessive flow. Thus, until body heat generation needs the skin of the arms and hands to dilate in order to dissipate warmth, these areas may turn cool and the fingers may tingle.

"Claudication" applies to the crampy discomfort that can progress to severe pain that is caused by inadequate blood supply to muscles of the exercising leg or arm. The term "intermittent" often precedes "claudication" because the pain is characteristically produced only by activity and relieved by rest.

Many studies have documented a prolongation in the time until onset of discomfort (or Grade 3 pain) as a result of an exercise program. The optimum schedule for such improvement, however, has not been established. Clinical impressions support the idea that walking or bicycle riding, twice daily and at least five days a week, will provide good results if undertaken with intelligent regard for weather and the terrain covered. The intensity of effort should permit a gradual warm-up and not elicit more than a Grade 2 discomfort. This takes a bit of "trial-and-error" practice.

Within the recommended minimum walking period of 20 minutes, many patients find a "warm-up" or "walk-through" capability that permits a faster pace without increased discomfort. Continued walking for at least 10 minutes after such a readjustment appears to be a reasonable approach. This effect may take longer in cold weather or after a meal.

The major cause of poor circulation to the extremities is atherosclerotic deposition of the same type that impairs coronary circulation. Thus, those individuals with coronary disease are more likely to have peripheral vascular disorders, and vice versa. It is important, therefore, to be sure that as the patients improve their walking capability they do not overtax their coronary circulation. Electrocardiographic monitoring every four to six months during a treadmill walking evaluation will help avoid undetected coronary insufficiency. As patients feel reassured with their lessening leg pain, we must ask them about chest discomfort as well.

Cramping that occurs in the calf muscles alone is often helped by a bicycle exercise program with the pedals under the instep of a strongly supported shoe rather than under the ball of the foot. More total leg and total body exercises can be achieved this way because the gastrocnemius muscles are spared the "push-off" demands of walking, jogging, and running. Some claudicators can learn to jog with a short stride but it is not easily done. Swimming is excellent exercise, of course, but should be done in shallow water so that if a cramp occurs it can be pushed out against the bottom. It is important to include a prolonged cool-down after exercise, particularly if discomfort was elicited. This helps prevent the buildup of residual metabolic products that may lead to further cramping.

VARICOSE VEINS. Clinical observations suggest that an increase in habitual physical activity may produce a diminuition in the size, appearance, and dysfunctional characteristics of varicose veins. Unfortunately, no controlled studies are known. Support hose helps but is hot and may be uncomfortable.

Kilbom has shown that bicycle exercise diminishes afternoon lower leg swelling in women who have minimal or no venous disease. The mechanism involved, however, may not involve changes in venomotor tone. It is considered likely that physical activity valued for other health reasons will also help prevent thrombophlebitis.

PROGRAMS FOR OTHER CARDIOVASCULAR DISEASES

With regard to other cardiovascular diseases, space does not permit inclusion of more than a few additional comments. Each patient needs specific counselling relative to individual features of a particular disease and often frequent revisions.

ARTERIAL HYPERTENSION. As mentioned in Section 1, there is evidence to suggest that a physical activity program may reduce the medication needed to control high blood pressure. From our understanding of the disturbed physiology (pathophysiology) of hypertension, exercise appears most beneficial when *frequency* and *duration* are emphasized rather than *intensity*. At least a 20-minute daily activity period, including 10 minutes of active perspiration, appears most likely to help break the increased arteriolar tone that causes the high resistance and resulting increased pressure. Exercise before lunch or dinner is preferred over early in the morning. This helps curb the appetite and reduce the accumulated tensions of the day. While perspiration is suggested to obtain maximal vasodilation to the skin, overdressing in cold weather is not recommended. Plastic or other nonbreathing clothing is always considered inappropriate and can be hazardous. Many people feel that swimming produces a superior sense of relaxation that may compensate for the lack of skin vasodilation in cool water.

Isometric or near isometric forms of exercise, such as water skiing, are not recommended. These activities produce further increases in blood pressure. If bicycling is included, a purposeful effort should be made to decrease arm tension and hand grip. Smooth running and swinging or rhythmical type sports like tennis may be superior to the more rapid muscular efforts of handball. For all activities, a prolonged warm-up is desirable. Individual adjustments in the exercise prescription are needed. The results from an exercise tolerance test will guide the hypertensive patient as to the best level of activity (intensity).

It is helpful if hypertensive patients have a record of blood pressure measurements to present to their physician for adjustment of activity, medications, and other life-style components. They may need more than standard constraints on consumption of alcohol, coffee, cola, and other stimulating beverages. Certainly tobacco use should be discontinued.

For persons who are interested in more specific details concerning cardiac rehabilitation, see Appendix C. It provides a discussion on other special problems that deal with the heart patient, for example, pulmonary hypertension, assymetric septal hypertrophy, atrioventricular heart block, and mitral valve prolapse, as well as three case studies of different diseases and complications.

SUMMARY

Increasing acceptance of the importance of cardiac rehabilitation has brought educational and personally prescribed exercise programs into many hospitals and has stimulated valuable developments in community facilities such as YMCA's and Jewish Community Centers. More adequate support of these and other well-structured efforts as an integral part of the optimal treatment of cardiovascular disease is still needed, particularly by the health insurance programs. Predictable physiologic and psychologic improvement is almost universally appreciated by both patients and staff and has been documented by careful research. The cost effectiveness of such efforts relative to increased productivity and decreased morbidity and mortality has not been adequately studied yet.

The most important lesson from the experience of the last two decades is that the majority of post-heart attack rehabilitation efforts result in the achievement of a full capability to live a meaningful and active life.

REFERENCES

1. American Heart Association Committee on Exercise. *Exercise testing and training of individuals with heart disease or at risk*

of its development, a handbook for physicians. 1975.

2. Barnes, G.K., M.J. Ray, A. Oberman, and N.T. Kouchoukos. "Changes in working status of patients following coronary bypass surgery." *JAMA, 238,* 1259-1262 (1977).

3. Cardiac Rehabilitation 1975. "Report of a joint working party of the Royal College of Physicians of London and the British Cardiac Society." *J. Royal Coll. of Phys.,* London, *9,* 281-346 (1975).

4. Conrad, C.C., et al. "How different sports rate in promoting physical fitness." *Medical Times, 104,* 65-72 (1976).

5. Donaldson, R., *Guidelines for Successful Jogging.* National Jogging Association, 1910 K St. N.W. Washington, D.C. 1977.

6. Fletcher, G.C., and J.D. Cantwell. *Exercise and Coronary Heart Disease,* C. Thomas, Springfield, 1974.

7. Fox, S.M. (ed.). *Coronary Heart Disease—Prevention, Detection Rehabilitation with Emphasis on Exercise Testing.* International Medical Corp., Denver, 1974.

8. Gentry, W.D., and R.B. Williams, (eds.). *Psychological Aspects of Myocardial Infarction and Coronary Care.* C.V. Mosby Co., St. Louis, 1975.

9. American College of Sports Medicine, *Guidelines For Graded Exercise Testing & Exercise Prescription.* Lea & Febiger, Philadelphia, 1975.

10. Harpur, J.E., W.T. Conner, M. Hamilton, R.J. Keller, H.J.B. Galbraith, J.J. Murray, and G.A. Rose. "Controlled trial of early mobilization and discharge from the hospital in uncomplicated myocardial infarction." *Lancet, 2,* 1331 (1971).

11. Hellerstein, H.K., and E.H. Friedman. "Sexual activity and the post-coronary patient." *Med. Asp. Human Sex, 3,* 70 (1969).

12. Kasch, F.W., "Choosing an activity." *Physician and Sports Med, 5,* 105 (1977).

13. Kellermann, J.J. and H. Denolin (eds.). *Critical Evaluation of Cardiac Rehabilitation.* S. Karger, New York, 1977.

14. Levine, S.A., and B. Lown. "Armchair treatment of acute coronary thrombosis." *JAMA, 148,* 1365 (1952).

15. Mallory, G.K., P.D., White, J. Salcedo-Salger, The speed of healing

of myocardial infarction. American Heart Journal, *18*:647, 1939.

16. Manninen V. & P. Halonen, Eds. Physical activity and coronary heart disease. Advances in Cardiology, Vol 18, 1976. S. Karger, New York.

17. Markiewicz, W., N. Houston and R.F. DeBusk, Exercise testing soon after myocardial infarction, Circ *56*:26-31, 1977.

18. Myocardial Infarction: How to prevent, how to rehabilitate. Council on Rehabilitation, International Society of Cardiology, Geneva, 1973.

19. Naughton, J.P., H.K. Hellerstein & L.C. Mohler, Eds. Exercise Testing and Exercise Training in Coronary Heart Disease, Academic Press, 1973. New York.

20. Needs and opportunities for rehabilitating the coronary heart disease patient. Report of the Task Force on Cardiovascular Rehabilitation of the National Heart and Lung Institute, 1974. DHEW Publ. #(NIH) 75-750. NIH, Bethesda, M. 20014.

21. Physical Fitness/Sports Medicine, a quarterly recurring bibliography, Superintendent of Documents, Government Printing Office, Washington DC 20402.

22. Sanne, H., D. Elmfeldt & L. Wilhelmsen, Preventive effect of physical training after a myocardial infarction, in Tibblin G, Keys A & Werko L, Eds. Preventive Cardiology 154-160, 1972, John Wiley & Sons, New York.

23. Stein, R.A., The effect of exercise training on heart rate during coitus in the post myocardial infarction patient, Circulation *55*, 735-740, 1977.

24. Stocksmeier, U., Ed, Psychological Approach to the Rehabilitation of Coronary Patients, 1976, Springer-Verlag, New York.

25. Wanka, J., Bedpan vs. commode in patients with myocardial infarction. Cardiac Rehabilitation *1*:7, 1970.

26. Wenger, N.K., C.A. Gilbert & N. Skorapa, Cardiac conditioning after myocardial infarction. An early intervention program. Cardiac Rehabilitation *2*:17, 1971.

27. Wenger, N.K., Rehabilitation after myocardial infarction, American Heart Association, Dallas, 1973.

28. Wilson, P.K., Ed. Adult Fitness and Cardiac Rehabilitation, University Park Press, Baltimore, 1975.

29. Zohman, L.R., R.E. Phillips, Progress in Rehabilitation, Medical Aspects of Exercise Testing and Training, 1973, Intercontinental Medical Book Corp., New York.

Section 6

Nutritional Aspects of Human Performance

INTRODUCTION

An ergogenic aid has been defined by Morgan as a substance or phenomena that elevates or improves the performance of an individual above normal expectations. Coaches and athletes alike are continuously searching for that slight edge that might assure victory and delay defeat. For some athletes, a special diet might be the deciding factor, others might rely on altering psychological states, while still others may try various hormones or pharmacological agents. Although there are obvious substances and phenomena that are truly ergogenic in nature, that is, they do facilitate performance, of what value is nutrition in improving performance? Do such practices as carbohydrate loading, megavitamin supplementation, and high protein intake actually influence athletic performance under controlled conditions? Do buffalo meat, dessicated liver, vitamins A, C, and E, or honey actually accomplish what has been claimed by various prominent athletes? Is performance enhanced? Unfortunately, this is an area that has been contaminated with individual bias, traditional beliefs and practices, and superstition.

To date, the most common conclusion drawn by the various authors who have investigated the role of nutrition in athletics is that a well-balanced diet is all that is necessary to insure optimal performance. Much of the available research literature is in direct conflict, that is, for every study demonstrating an ergogenic effect for a certain food, vitamin, or mineral, there is another study that demonstrates no significant effect. The purpose of this review is to briefly summarize what is currently known about nutrition as an ergogenic aid, concentrating on the most recent research. While much of the claim for certain foods or substances can be attributed to the psychological effect, that is, one expects a particular food to aid performance, evidence is mounting that there are certain nutritional manipulations that can improve the athlete's performance.

NUTRITIONAL SUPPLEMENTS OR MANIPULATIONS

Here we focus on the various foods and substances that have typically been used by athletes to enhance or facilitate performance. Many foods, vitamins, and minerals will not be discussed either because they have never been used or claimed as ergogenic aids, or there is little or no research available to support or refute the ergogenic aid properties of the food or substance. Often, one of the important limitations to many investigations dealing with the effect that supplementations and various dietary manipulations have on performance is the lack of a good control group. If the experimental subject is administered a supplement that is supposed to enhance performance, it is very likely that improvements will be shown. The question is, was the improvement purely physiological or, because of the power of suggestion, psychological? To avoid the possible psychological effect, experiments should be conducted double blind, whereby neither the subjects (control or experimental) or investigator know who is getting the actual supplement. In this case, the control subject will be administered the same color pill (or whatever) and not know that it has no nutritional value.

PROTEIN. Is it necessary for the athlete who is in training for the purpose of increasing strength and muscle bulk to supplement his or her normal dietary intake of protein? Protein is essential for the growth and development of the various tissues of the body. It has been thought for many years that proteins had to be supplemented in rather liberal quantities. In fact, at one time, it was thought that the muscle consumed itself as fuel for its own muscular contraction, and that protein supplementation was essential to prevent the muscles from being totally consumed. This practice was first recorded in Greece during the 5th century B.C. It is now recognized that little protein is consumed as fuel for muscular work. If fats or carbohydrates are available, they are selected preferentially over proteins as the source of energy.

Studies have shown that work performance is neither enhanced nor inhibited by protein supplementation or deprivation. In a recent study, two groups of young men consumed two levels of protein (1.4 and 2.8 grams per kilogram body weight) during a 40-day experimental period of heavy physical activity. It was found that the group receiving the low protein intake was receiving adequate protein to maintain nitrogen (protein) equilibrium. However, the men on the high protein diet did increase body protein stores and muscle mass with high protein diets. In studies investigating the ergogenic properties of anabolic steroids, it does appear that the steroids do facilitate gains in lean body weight and performance, but only when a protein supplement is provided with the steroid. Thus, from the above, it does appear that protein might facilitate the growth of lean tissue, but whether this translates into an increase in performance remains to be established.

FAT AND CARBOHYDRATE. In the not too distant past, carbohydrate was regarded as the major fuel for muscular contraction. It is now realized that fat is a major, if not the most importance source of fuel for light to moderate levels of activity. However, this does not imply that the athlete should attempt to store more body fat, since he or she is already storing more than will ever be needed. A pound or two of fat is sufficient to provide the total energy needed for a grueling 26.2 mile, 3 hour marathon run. A theory has been proposed that the higher levels of fat found in women provide them with an advantage in long distance races, but this has yet to be proven. Therefore, fat is not considered to have any special ergogenic properties. In fact, extra fat weight that has to be carried by a runner can be considered dead weight and will be detrimental to performance.

One of the biggest breakthroughs in athletic nutrition came in the 1960's when a group of Scandinavian researchers started experimental observations of carbohydrate storage and utilization with prolonged endurance type exercise. Use of the needle biopsy technique (a long, thick needle type device that samples a small piece of muscle) for muscle sampling and a number of new micromethods for the determination of substrate and intermediary metabolite concentrations (cellular function of muscular work) provided major advances in our understanding of the nutrition of athletic performance. Earlier work had suggested that carbohydrate supplementation would facilitate endurance performance. This was confirmed by the finding that exhaustion from endurance exercise was always accompanied by hypoglycemia or low blood sugar. In addition, it was found that when working at or above 85 to 90 percent of maximum oxygen uptake, the total source of energy was derived from carbohydrates. Hence, it became obvious by the 1960's that carbohydrates were not only an important fuel source but also, by supplementing carbohydrates in the diet, it was possible to improve endurance performance.

By taking serial muscle biopsies at consecutive, fixed time intervals during endurance exercise, it has been shown that the muscle glycogen (carbohydrate-sugar) content decreases as work is prolonged (see Figure 6.1) and that muscle glycogen stores can become totally depleted, which coincides with the attainment of muscular exhaustion. It has also been shown that the initial glycogen content of the muscle is critical to prolonged exercise, that is, the greater the initial glycogen content, the longer the individual can perform (see Figure 6.2). From Figure 6.2 it is also apparent that the composition of the diet prior to the performance is critical to determining the initial levels of glycogen in the muscle, and therefore is critical to the performance itself.

Bergström and associates investigated this aspect of performance enhancement in 1967. Each of their subjects was given three different diets, each for a prescribed period of time. One diet was high in carbohydrate, one high in fat and protein, and one was a normal mixed diet. Each diet contained the same number of calories. Before starting the diet, the subjects depleted their muscle glycogen stores by riding a bicycle ergometer to exhaustion at approximately 75 percent of their maximal oxygen uptake. This was followed by three days on the prescribed diet and then a second ride to exhaustion. Prior to the second ride, a muscle biopsy was obtained to determine the initial glycogen content. The total length of time the subject could ride before reaching exhaustion and the initial glycogen content of the active muscles were as follows.

DIET	GLYCOGEN CONTENT (grams per 100 grams of wet tissue)	RIDING TIME TO EXHAUSTION (minutes)
Mixed	1.93	125.8
High fat and protein	0.69	58.8
High carbohydrate	3.70	189.3

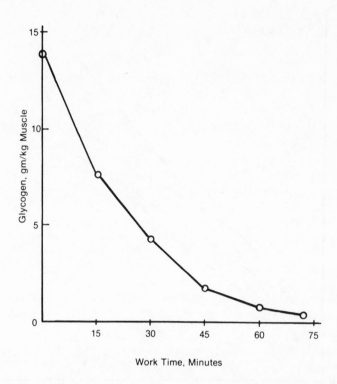

FIGURE 6.1. Glycogen content in the quadriceps muscle during intermittent bicycle work. (Courtesy of Bergström and Hultman.)

These results support the conclusion that endurance performance can be significantly altered by manipulating the diet, in this case by loading up on carbohydrates before competition to enhance the glycogen stores.

A practical example of this same phenomenon was shown in an experiment in which the subjects each participated in two 30 kilometer races, one with a high carbohydrate diet following muscle glycogen depletion, and one with a normal, mixed diet. The average muscle glycogen content was elevated on the high carbohydrate diet to nearly double the level attained on the mixed diet. In addition, the 30 kilometer race times were substantially faster following the high carbohydrate diet, the improvement coming primarily in the last half of

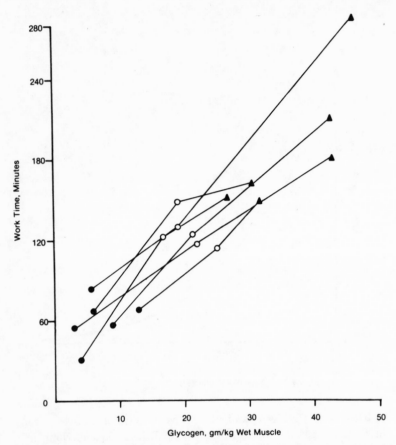

FIGURE 6.2. Relation between initial glycogen content in quadriceps femoris and work time in six subjects on a bicycle ergometer with the same relative work load; three times each with three-day interval. Diets before exercise: ○ mixed; ● carbohydrate-free; and ▲ carbohydrate-rich. (Courtesy of Bergström and Hultman.)

the race.

With this available information, how does the athlete proceed to enhance his or her muscle glycogen stores to increase performance? First, carbohydrates are normally stored in limited quantities, and only a limited quantity of carbohydrate can be absorbed from the intestine during the actual competition; thus, it is necessary to enlarge the glycogen stores. To increase glycogen storage, the individual must first deplete his or her glycogen stores. This can be accomplished by an exhaustive exercise bout of an extended duration, that is, greater than 60 to 90 minutes. This should be done approximately seven days before the competition. The greater the depletion, the greater can be the additional storage of glycogen. Once depleted, the glycogen stores are maintained in this depleted state by continued training and a low-carbohydrate diet. A certain amount of carbohydrate is essential, so the diet should not be totally void of carbohydrate. Approximately three to four days prior to competition, the diet is changed to one that is predominantly carbohydrate. Additional fluids must also be ingested, since 3 to 4 grams of water are stored with each gram of glycogen. While on the high carbohydrate diet, activity should be tapered to low levels to maximize the additional storage of glycogen.

A possible warning must be sounded to those who advocate this type of dietary manipulation. Several physicians have become concerned about the possibility of medical risks associated with this kind of dietary practice. Angina like symptoms (chest pain) have been noted in several athletes who have used this diet. In one case, this was associated with an abnormal electrocardiogram. It is not possible, at the present time, to establish a cause-effect relationship. It seems unlikely that carbohydrate loading would be dangerous to the young, healthy athlete. It might be wise for the older athlete to proceed with caution, however, until this phenomenon is better understood. Most endurance athletes are unknowlingly practicing carbohydrate loading to a great extent just by the nature of their rigorous training programs. Although they might not go through a three- to four -day extensive reduction in carbohydrate intake following an exhaustive, glycogen depleting workout, they do periodically deplete their glycogen stores and consume considerable quantities of carbohydrates.

Carbohydrate loading increases the total quantity of glycogen available in the muscle. How does this, in itself, improve performance? During prolonged endurance competition when the body depletes its carbohydrate stores, the body cannot perform equally well by using fat as the main source of fuel. A number of studies have now shown conclusively that while fat is a major source of fuel for low intensity exercise up to 70 percent of maximal oxygen uptake, that, as the intensity of the exercise increases, the reliance on carbohydrates increases. Once the anaerobic threshold (non-oxidative metabolism) is reached and the oxygen supply is unable to meet the oxygen demands, the body shifts to a dependence on carbohydrate utilization. Horstman, in his review of athletic nutrition, has provided insight into why this shift occurs. In calculating the actual energy production from a given fuel, it is possible to calculate the efficiency of utilization. This is defined simply as the calories of energy produced per minute from a specific fuel per liter of oxygen consumed, or the energy derived per liter of oxygen. Glucose yields 5.01 calories per liter of oxygen, and fat yields only 4.65 calories per liter of oxygen. This provides a distinct advantage for carbohydrate utilization when the exercise intensity reaches the upper levels, since there is a greater energy yield for the same amount of oxygen consumed.

VITAMINS AND MINERALS. Historically, massive doses of various vitamins and minerals have been taken by certain athletes with the hope of improving their athletic performance. The many health problems and diseases associated with various vitamin deficiencies are well known, but do athletes generally have vitamin or mineral deficiencies? Even if deficiencies do not exist, will supplementation of any one vitamin or mineral above the recommended daily dose result in a better performance? Although these questions have been researched extensively, debate still continues over the conflicting results.

B-complex vitamins are among those vitamins known to influence physical performance. They are involved in coenzyme activity with the metabolism of fats and carbohydrates. Deficiencies have been shown to decrease athletic performance. On the other hand, supplementation of B-complex vitamins, primarily thiamine (B_1), has been shown to both improve performance as well as to have no influence on performance. Additional research is needed to provide a conclusive answer to the question of whether B-complex supplementation is of any value for the athlete.

Vitamin C also plays an important role in energy metabolism. Similiar to a deficiency in the B vitamins, a deficiency in vitamin C will result in a decrease in physical performance. With regard to the question of supplementation, the research literature is again controversial. Early studies of vitamin C supplementation and physical performance showed no distinct advantage in consuming levels of vitamin C in excess of the recommended daily dosage. More recent studies, however, have reopened interest in this area. A number of studies conducted since

1960 have shown vitamin C supplementation to result in prolonged endurance capacity. These recent findings point to the need for additional studies to clarify the role of vitamin C in endurance performance relative to its mechanism of operation and to the optimal dosage.

Vitamin E must be considered the wonder vitamin of this century, since it has been touted as the cure for almost all of our illnesses. As with the vitamins discussed above, the research literature relative to the influences of vitamin E on athletic performance is in conflict. Using wheat germ oil, a rich source of alpha tocopherol and a most potent source of vitamin E, several studies have shown improvements in endurance performance, while several others have shown little or no effect from the vitamin. Again the evidence must be considered inconclusive at this time, indicating the need for further study of a highly controlled nature.

From the above studies, it would appear that the B-complex vitamins and vitamins C and E may have ergogenic properties, but this conclusion is certainly open to debate. Additional studies are essential, since vitamin supplementation is expensive and can even be toxic as in the case of the fat soluble vitamins, that is, A, D, E, and K, which are stored in the body. Since, the water soluble vitamins are rapidly excreted in the urine, supplementation of these vitamins, if they have no measurable effect on performance, leaves the athlete with nothing more than expensive urine.

With minerals, it is well known that deficiencies can reduce the efficiency of the athlete, particularly when exercising in the heat. Sweating reduces the body's sodium and chloride stores. In addition, exercise can substantially alter the body's balance for potassium, calcium, magnesium, and phosphorus. Again, as in the above discussion of vitamins, it is essential to replace those minerals that have been lost, but is supplementation above normal levels an aid to performance?

The use of salt tablets has been advocated for years to supplement the normal salt ingested in food when the athlete is exercising under conditions where there is excessive water and mineral loss through sweating. While replacement of sodium chloride lost in sweat is desirable, care must be taken not to ingest more salt than is necessary. Excessive salt intake can lead to undesirable potassium loss and increased water retention, and be dangerous for persons with high blood pressure. Generally, according to most review articles, a liberal salting of food or the ingestion of an electrolyte solution such as Gatorade,

Sportade, ERG, or other similar, readily available commercial beverages, is sufficient to maintain sodium and chloride levels, without having to ingest salt tablets. Caution should be exercised concerning the use of the commercially prepared supplemental fluid and electrolyte aids though, because many are too high in sugar content. Too high a sugar content can lead to a slight body dehydration as a result of body water absorbing back into the stomach to help dilute the highly concentrated fluid. A highly concentrated fluid also slows down the absorption process in the small intestine. The problem can be eliminated by diluting the solutions with water.

Aspartates have been used as ergogenic aids for a number of years. Aspartates are potassium and magnesium salts of aspartic acid, which supposedly work in an intermediate position in the Krebs cycle (oxygen utilization) to reduce the accumulation of blood ammonia. Increased levels of blood ammonia are thought to be one possible cause of fatigue; thus, aspartates are considered to have possible ergogenic effects by delaying the onset of fatigue. Several studies of a well designed and controlled nature demonstrated rather remarkable gains in endurance from aspartate administration, but several others have shown aspartates to have no influence. Again, additional research is needed to clarify the actual role, or aspartates in prolonging activities of an indurance nature.

WATER. Seldom is water regarded as an ergogenic aid. It is consumed by everyone, has no caloric or nutritional benefits, but is essential to life. From Costill's extensive review of the literature, it appears that water is an ergogenic aid. Ingesting fluids prior to endurance competition is an effective way to maintain the body temperature at a reduced level and to limit the extent of dehydration. See Section 7 for more specific recommendations for water ingestion in relation to heat and endurance performance.

PRECONTEST MEAL. For years, the athlete has been given the traditional steak dinner several hours prior to competition. Possibly, this practice originated from the early belief that the muscle consumed itself as fuel for muscular activity, and steak provided the necessary protein to counteract this loss. It is now recognized that this is probably the worst possible meal that the athlete could eat prior to competition. Steak contains a high percentage of fat, which takes many hours to be fully digested. The digestive process competes for the available blood with the muscles that are used in the contest. Therefore, no matter what its content, the precontest meal should be given no later than three hours before the contest. Another factor to consider is the emo-'ional climate at the time of this meal. Extreme nervousness is frequently present, and even the choicest steak is not enjoyed. The steak would be psychologically more satisfying to the athlete the night before the contest.

Many athletes are starting to use a liquid pregame meal, since it is palatable, digests relatively easily, and is less likely to result in nervous indigestion, nausea, vomiting, and abdominal cramps. Those who have experimented with the liquid precontest meals have found them to be highly satisfactory. Presently, this would appear to be the best available choice as a pregame meal.

SUMMARY

One of the areas receiving greatest attention and interest among athletes relative to improved athletic performance is nutrition. Can a person alter what he or she eats to improve performance? Although it appears that the average athlete consumes a sufficient quantity of protein, supplementation may have a limited effect on gains in lean weight. Carbohydrate supplementation or loading is an effective nutritional manipulative technique that can increase general muscular endurance by increasing the storage of muscle glycogen. Various vitamins and minerals have been proposed as ergogenic aids. From the available research, it appears that vitamins B_1, C, and E may have ergogenic properties, but the available evidence is not conclusive. Aspartates have also been proposed as ergogenic aids, but again, the research literature is equivocal. Water, while generally not considered as an ergogenic aid, definitely has ergogenic properties. Last, the use of an appropriate pregame meal was discussed, and it was suggested that a liquid pregame meal has many benefits for athletes in all sports.

In conclusion, there is far more information to be gained than what presently exists in the area of nutritional manipulation to improve athletic performance. There is a critical need to initiate additional studies in each of these areas because past research has had conflicting results.

REFERENCES

1. Bergström, J., R.C. Harris, E. Hultman, et al. "Energy-rich phos-

phagens in dynamic and static work. " *Advances Exp. Med. Biol.*, *11*:341-355 (1971).

2. Bergström, J., L. Hermansen, E. Hultman, and B. Saltin. "Diet, muscle, glycogen, and physical performance." *Acta. Physiol. Scand.*, *71*:140-150 (1967).

3. Bergström, J., and E. Hultman. "Muscle glycogen synthesis after exercise: An enhancing factor localized to the muscle cells in man." *Nature, 210*:309-310 (1966).

4. Bergström, J., and E. Hultman. "Nutrition for maximum sports performance." *JAMA, 221*:999-1006 (1972).

5. Christensen, E.H., and O. Hansen, III. "Arbeits fähigkeit ünd Erna hrung." *Scand. Arch. Physiol., 81*:160-171 (1939).

6. Christophe, J., and J. Mayer. "Effect of exercise on glucose uptake in rats and men." *J. Appl. Physiol., 13*:269-272 (1958).

7. Consolazio, C.F., H.L. Johnson, R.A. Nelson, J.G. Dramise, and J.H. Skala. "Protein metabolism during intensive physical training in the young adult." *Amer. J. Clin. Nutr., 38*:29-35 (1975).

8. Costill, D.L., "Water and electrolytes." In: *Ergogenic Aids and Muscular Performance*, W.P. Morgan (ed.). New York: Academic Press, 1972, pp. 293-318.

9. Frankau, I.M. "Acceleration of co-ordinated muscular effort by nicotinamide. Preliminary report to the Medical Research Council." *Brit. Med. J., 2*:601-603 (1943).

10. Horstman, D.H. "Nutrition." In: *Ergogenic Aids and Muscular Performance*, W.P. Morgan (ed.) New York: Academic Press, 1972, pp. 343-363.

11. Howald, H., B. Segesser, and W.F. Körner. "Ascorbic acid and athletic performance." *Ann. NY Acad. Sci., 258*:458-464 (1975).

12. Hultman, E. "Studies on muscle metabolism of glycogen and active phosphate in man with special reference to exercise and diet." *Scand. J. Clin. Lab. Invest., 19* Suppl. *94*:1-63 (1967).

13. Karlsson, J., and B. Saltin. "Diet, muscle glycogen, and endurance performance." *J. Appl. Physiol., 31*:203-206 (1971).

14. Keys, A. "Physical performance in relation to diet." *Fed. Proc.*

Fed. Amer. Soc. Exp. Biol., 2:164-187 (1943).

15. Keys, A., and A.F. Henschel. "Vitamin supplementation of U.S. Army rations in relation to fatigue and the ability to do muscular work." *J. Nutr., 23*:259-269 (1942).

16. Keys, A., and A.F. Henschel, O. Mickelsen, and J. Brožek. "The performance of normal young men on controlled thiamine intakes." *J. Nutr., 26*:399-415 (1943).

17. Londeree, B. "Pre-event diet routine." *Runner's World, 9*:26-29 (1974).

18. Mayer, J., and B. Bullen. "Nutrition and athletic performance." *Physiol. Rev., 40*:369-397 (1960).

19. Morgan, W.P. *Preface to Ergogenic Aids and Muscular Performance,* W.P. Morgan (ed.). New York: Academic Press, 1972.

20. Nyhan. W.L., A.O. Yujnovsky, and R.F. Wehr. "Amino acids and cell growth." In: *Human Growth: Body Composition, Cell Growth, Energy and Intelligence,* D.B. Cheek (ed.). Philadelphia: Lea and Febiger, 1968.

21. Parizkova, J. "Nutrition, body fat and physical fitness." *Bordon Review of Nutrition Research, 29*:41-54 (1968).

22. Simonson, E., N. Enzer, A. Baer, and R. Braun. "The influence of vitamin B (complex) surplus on the capacity for muscular and mental work." *J. Ind. Hyg. Toxicol., 24*:83-90 (1942).

23. Smith, N.J. *Food for Sport.* Palo Alto, CA: Bull Publishing, 1976.

24; Van Huss, W.D. "What made the Russians run?" *Nutr. Today, 1*:20-23 (1966).

25. Williams M.H. *Nutritional Aspects of Human Physical and Athletic Performance.* Springfield, Ill.: C.C. Thomas, 1976.

Section 7
Special Considerations

INTRODUCTION

Once the commitment has been made to begin an exercise program, attention must be given to a number of factors that can directly influence the program's success or failure. What type of clothing should be worn when exercising, and how important is proper footwear? What steps can be followed to minimize the possibility of serious orthopedic injury? Is warm-up necessary, and what is the proper way in which to cool down following a bout of vigorous exercise? How does altitude or extreme variations in temperature and humidity influence the daily workout? Does one's age or sex become factors in modifying the exercise program, or limit the degree of improvement that might be expected to result from the exercise program? Can the exercise prescription be followed when traveling, or when forced inside during inclement weather? How does one stay motivated to continue his or her exercise program from day to day, or year to year? These and many other questions of a similar nature will be discussed in this section.

CLOTHING, SHOES, AND SPECIAL EQUIPMENT

The selection of improper or inappropriate clothing, shoes, or related equipment can create many problems for the neophyte who is just beginning his or her exercise program. Overdressing or underdressing, wearing the wrong size or type of shoe, or using the wrong piece of equipment can lead to serious problems of heat or cold stress, disability, injury, overstress, or an unnecessary expense.

CLOTHING. The choice of clothing will be totally dependent on the specific activity selected and the environmental conditions under which the activity will be performed. With swimming, the conditions are relatively stable throughout the year and, as a result, special considerations are not required when selecting a swimming suit. For hiking, walking, jogging, running, bicycling, or any other sporting activity that is performed outdoors, the appropriate attire should be comfortable, reasonably loose, and of the proper weight to insure protection from the sun, cold, and wind. As a general rule of thumb, it is better to underdress than overdress, since the exercise itself will have a considerable warming effect on the body. Women should avoid restrictive support garments or clothing that would impede movement or blood flow. Bras may or may not be worn depending on the size of the breasts. It is generally felt that a bra is beneficial for women with large breasts. Although men should wear supporters when participating in vigorous sports, supporters are not essential during an activity such as jogging and may lead to skin irritations during long periods of activity.

Although there is a great deal of individual variation, the following suggestions should prove helpful. When exercising at temperatures between 60 to 80°F, a light T-shirt or blouse and shorts would be adequate; from 40 to 60°F, a sweat shirt is advisable, and for temperatures below 40°F, sweat pants and thermal underwear may be required. Gloves and stocking caps are also desirable when the temperature drops below 50°F. At temperatures above 80°F, men may wish to exercise without a shirt and women may elect to wear a halter top. These recommendations are made assuming that there are moderate levels of humidity and wind. With higher humidities, the extreme high and low temperatures are considerably more stressful. Direct radiation from the sun is also an important consideration.

Under no circumstances should one exercise while wearing rubberized or plastic clothing. This is common practice among individuals who are trying to use exercise as a means of losing weight. Athletes such as jockeys and wrestlers frequently use this technique to get down to their prescribed weight limit. The increased sweat loss does not result in a permanent loss of body weight, and this practice can be very dangerous. The rubberized or plastic clothing does not allow the body sweat to evaporate. Since this is the principle manner in which the body regulates its temperature during exercise, it can lead to a dramatic increase in body temperature, excessive dehydration and salt loss, and possible heat stroke or heat exhaustion.

SHOES AND SOCKS. The type of shoe selected and the proper fit of the shoe are important considerations for any activity program. For most activities, a good quality, well fitting tennis, basketball or general gym shoe is perfectly adequate. For jogging or running activities, however, a special and carefully fitted shoe designed specifically for these activities is highly recommended, since the foot strikes the ground, supporting the majority of the body weight, many times during a single workout. This places considerable stress on the foot and its associated structures. Thus, a shoe that gives good support and protection and has shock absorbing qualities is highly desirable. Most of the better running shoes have a strong, highly supportive heel cup, a heel wedge, good arch support, a comfortable innersole, and a relatively pliable outer sole. Prices will vary between $20.00 and $40.00 for a pair of the better rated shoes. *Runner's World*, a monthly publication for runners of both sexes, all ages, and all abilities (from the beginning jogger to the world-class runner), devotes one issue annually (September) to rating the various running shoes. See this magazine for a listing of the top rated running shoes.

Socks are also important items for the beginning exerciser. Wool or cotton socks are appropriate providing they fit properly following washing. Tube socks have become quite popular for they fit a variety of sizes, do not shrink appreciably, and tend to stay fixed to the foot. This latter point is important since creeping socks tend to bunch up and cause painful blisters.

SPECIAL EQUIPMENT. An activity such as swimming or jogging requires no special equipment other than that described above. If, however, the exercise prescription specifies games like tennis or racketball, or an indoor exercise device such as a stationary bicycle, proper knowledge of the equipment under consideration is important. It would be impos-

discuss here all possible items of equipment likely to be used in
rcise program designed to promote cardiorespiratory fitness.
However, there are certain guidelines that can be applied in the purchase of most specialized exercise equipment, including the following.

o Deal with reputable businesses that will stand behind their products.

o Consult experts in the field or various consumer reports if there is
  any question about a company or its product. Most YMCAs, colleges,
  or universities have experts in this area that would be willing to provide valuable information. Also, the American College of Sports
  Medicine* will provide advice on request.

o Avoid devices that claim to do all of the work. Active participation is
  essential to obtain the desired benefits of exercise.

o Do not be misled into thinking that the more expensive the item, the
  better job it does. Many items of equipment are greatly overpriced.

o Do not buy something that will not be used. Many expensive items
  of exercise equipment end up being stored in the garage, basement,
  or attic.

o Do not buy on impulse after receiving a high powered sales pitch.
  Wait at least three days before making the final decision.

o Understand completely the purpose of the exercise device and its
  principle of operation.

WARM-UP, COOL-DOWN, AND INJURY PREVENTION

WARM-UP PERIOD. It is particularly important to incorporate a
brief, but basic warm-up routine into the endurance training program.
This was discussed briefly in Section 4, and appropriate stretching exercises were illustrated. The stretching exercises promote development
and maintenance of flexibility as well as preparing the muscles, joints,
and ligaments for the added stress of the cardiorespiratory endurance
training session. One study showed serious electrocardiogram abnormalities when sudden exercise was undertaken without proper warm-up.
Strength and muscular endurance exercises can be performed as a part
of the initial warm-up period, but they should be preceded by the
stretching exercises. If jogging (running), bicycling, hiking, and so on
are a participant's main endurance activity, then strength and muscular
endurance exercises should concentrate more on the upper body, be-

*American College of Sports Medicine, 1440 Monroe St. Madison, WI.

cause the lower body is the primary focus of these cardiorespiratory endurance programs. Proper warm-up will help alleviate many potential injuries such as muscle pulls, strains, sprains, and lower back discomfort, in addition to reducing the extent of muscle soreness.

COOL-DOWN PERIOD. The cool-down period is of equal importance. This is the period immediately following the cardiorespiratory endurance portion of each exercise session. The major purpose of the cool-down period is to keep the primary muscle groups, which were involved in the endurance exercise, continuously active. Since most cardiorespiratory endurance exercises involve the legs and are typically performed in an upright position, blood will pool in the lower half of the body if the individual does not perform light activity such as walking or slow jogging during the recovery period. This light activity allows the leg muscles to assist the return of the pooled blood to the heart. The blood travels from the heart to the leg muscles through arteries and returns to the heart through veins. A series of valves are located throughout the veins and permit blood to flow in only one direction, that is, back to the heart. As the muscles in the legs contract, they create pressure against the veins, which in turn pushes the blood toward the heart. Without this light activity, the blood will continue to pool in the lower body, and the participant may experience dizziness and can even pass out because of inadequate blood flow to the brain.

The light activity during the cool-down period also helps to prevent extreme muscle soreness. This is particularly true if the cool-down period includes a few selected stretching exercises that concentrate on the legs and lower back. The length of the cool-down period need not exceed 5 to 10 minutes. Following the workout, the participant should take a warm, *not hot*, shower, since hot showers following endurance exercise can create serious cardiovascular complications.

INJURY PREVENTION. The potential for serious injury exists in almost any exercise program if the proper precautions are not followed. Sudden vigorous exercise has been shown to place a potentially lethal strain on the heart. A proper warm-up period decreases the likelihood of this occurring. The participant must be aware of the various warning signs that may result from vigorous endurance exercise. Dr. Lenore Zohman, a prominant exercise cardiologist who has devoted many years to the study of exercise prescription for normal and cardiac patients, in her booklet, "Beyond Diet. . .Exercise your Way to Fitness and

Heart Health," has listed a number of potential warning signs and symptoms that could occur either during or immediately following exercise. These may be grouped into the following two categories.

A. *Stop Exercising.* See a physician before resuming:

1. Abnormal heart activity, including irregular pulse (missed beats or extra beats), fluttering, jumping or palpitations in the chest or throat, sudden burst of rapid heart beats, or a sudden slowing of a rapid pulse rate.

2. Pain or pressure in the center of the chest, or the arm or throat, during or immediately following exercise.

3. Dizziness, lightheadedness, sudden lack of coordination, confusion, cold sweating, glassy stare, pallor, blueness or fainting.

4. Illness, particularly viral infections, can lead to myocarditis, that is, viral infection of the heart muscle. Avoid exercise during and immediately following an illness.

B. *Attempt Self-Correction*

1. Persistent rapid pulse rate throughout 5 to 10 minutes of recovery or longer. *Self-Correction technique*: reduce intensity of the activity (use a lower training heart rate) and progress to higher levels of activity at a slower rate. Consult a physician if the condition persits.

2. Nausea or vomiting after exercise. *Self-Correction technique*: Reduce the intensity of the endurance exercise and prolong the cool-down period. Avoid eating for at least two hours prior to the exercise session.

3. Extreme breathlessness lasting more than 10 minutes after the cessation of exercise. *Self-Correction technique*: Reduce the intensity of the endurance exercise. Consult a physician if the condition persists.

4. Prolonged fatigue up to 24 hours following exercise. *Self-Correction technique*: Reduce the intensity of the endurance exercise and reduce the duration of the total workout session if this symptom persists. Consult a physician if these self-correcting techniques do not remedy the situation.

In addition to the above, there are a number of potential injuries or medical complications of an orthopedic nature that are usually minor, but can also result in many participants dropping out of their exercise programs. Dr. Brian J. Sharkey, Director of the Human Performance Laboratory at the University of Montana, has listed a number of these in his recent book, *Fitness and Work Capacity,* and has suggested a sound course of action to follow in an attempt to correct the situation. The list includes the following.

- *Blisters*—a common problem, particularly when breaking in a pair of new shoes. Prevention begins with properly fitting shoes, and socks that stay in place and do not creep or bunch up. When blisters occur, puncture the edge of the blister with a sterile needle, drain the fluid, apply a topical antiseptic, and cover with gauze or a Band-Aid. Use precaution to avoid possible infection.

- *Muscle soreness*— usually accompanies the start of any exercise program, or results from a sudden change in exercise habits, the exact cause of which is unknown. The degree of soreness can be reduced by starting at low levels of exercise and progressing slowly through the first few weeks, and by thorough warm-up and cool-down periods that include stretching exercises. Massage and warm baths help to relieve the soreness when present.

- *Muscle cramps*—involuntary muscle contractions that may be due to a salt and potassium imbalance in the muscle. Stretching and massaging the muscle usually brings immediate relief. Proper warm-up, replacement of salt and potassium lost through sweating, and post-exercise stretching should prevent most muscle cramps.

- *Bone bruises*—painful bruises, usually on bottoms of feet, caused by single blow or repeated trauma to the bone. Ice and padding of the bruised area provide some relief, but proper footwear, including good inner soles, usually prevents the problem.

- *Lower back pain*—usually the result of poor flexibility, weak abdominal and back muscles, and poor posture. Stretching and muscle strengthening exercises, with a conscious effort to improve posture, improves the problem in the majority of cases. The following exercises in Section 4 are designed specifically to prevent as well as to rehabilitate lower back problems: 1; 3a or 3b or 3c; 5a or 5b or 5c; 6; 7a or 7b or 7c; 10; 15a; 18a or 18b.

- *Knee problems*—can be caused or aggravated by the endurance conditioning program. This is a frequent area of complaint among joggers and runners. Wearing proper footwear and running on soft, even surfaces such as grass tend to reduce or eliminate the problem. Stay away from sharp turns. A physician or podiatrist should be consulted if the problem persists.

- *Shin splints*—a sharp pain on the front aspect of the shin bone (tibia). Shin splints are probably the result of a lowered arch, irritated membranes, tearing of muscle where it attaches to bone, hairline fracture of bone, or other factors. While rest is the only sure cure, limited exercise is possible with the leg wrapped or taped. Prevention of shin splints can be accomplished by proper footwear, running on soft surfaces such as grass, and strengthening the surrounding musculature. Refer to Exercises 7*A* or 7*B* or 7*C*, 9, 11*A* and 11*B* in Section 4 for appropriate stretching and strengthening exercises.

- *Achilles tendon injuries*—a frequent source of trouble in distance runners. Improper footwear, including shoes without heel wedges, and high back shoes that rub against the achilles tendon are considered to be the primary cause. Reduced activity or total rest combined with ice appear to be the only remedy. Prevention through selection of proper footwear and adequate warm-up are strongly advised. The warm-up should include a heal stretching exercise. See exercise 11*a* or 11*b*, Section 4.

- *Ankle Problems*—a frequent problem for those who play sports that require quick change in direction. A sprained ankle should be put in ice immediately to prevent major swelling and to facilitate recovery. Serious sprains should be examined by a physician. Prevention is best achieved by strengthening the surrounding musculature, wearing high topped gym or basketball shoes, and by preventive taping or ankle wraps.

If a jogger has an injury to the lower extremity and rest is required, he or she can use alternate activities such as cycling (stationary or free wheeling) or swimming. In this way general fitness can be maintained while the jogging injury has a chance to heel.

ENVIRONMENTAL CONSIDERATIONS

When exercising in a temperature controlled swimming pool or inside an air conditioned or heated building, the environment remains very stable from day to day and month to month, independent of changes in the outer environment. However, most individuals exercise outside of these controlled conditions, and factors such as heat, cold, humidity, and quality of air become major considerations. In addition, whether exercising under controlled conditions or not, any marked change in altitude will also significantly influence one's ability to exercise.

HEAT. The body's temperature is maintained very consistently at approximately 98.6°F under normal conditions. When confronted with variations in outside temperature, the body makes rather remarkable adjustments to maintain its temperature. When faced with extreme cold, the body shivers, which generates metabolic heat to maintain body temperature. In extreme heat, the body relies primarily on sweating to maintain a constant temperature. Sweating is effective only as long as the sweat can evaporate, since it is the evaporation of the sweat that cools the body. Wind also aids in the evaporative process. In very humid weather, since the air is saturated with water, evaporation becomes limited and thus the body has difficulty being cooled.

During exercise, the body temperature is maintained at a much higher level, from 100° to 104°F, which can be perfectly normal. From the standpoint of efficiency, the exercising body is more efficient at a higher body temperature. Exercise itself increases the heat production of the body as evidenced by the fact that when an individual is confronted with cold, moving around and keeping active helps that person stay warm.

The ability of an individual to successfully perform in a hot environment depends on the magnitude of heat, the existing humidity, the air movement, the intensity and duration of the exercise, and the extent of his or her previous exposure to heat (acclimatization). The amount of direct radiation is also a critical factor, for direct exposure to the sun, as opposed to shade or cloud cover, is a major source of heat gain through radiation.

The higher the temperature, the greater the heat stress on the individual. With low humidity, the individual can tolerate air temperatures in excess of 90°F without too much trouble, since the individual can sweat at rates in excess of 2 liters (approximately 2 quarts) per hour, and the dry air can evaporate most of the sweat. As the humidity increases, the tolerable heat level reduces considerably. In a dry climate the individual is not even aware he or she is sweating, since the sweat

..tes immediately the moment it reaches the skin. Under condi-
..f high humidity, the individual is quite conscious of sweating,
sin.. very little is being absorbed by the already saturated air, and the
sweat rolls off unceasingly. Another factor that is critical to determining the total stress is air movement. The greater the air movement
the greater the cooling effect. Still air stagnates, becomes saturated
with water, and evaporation is restricted.

The intensity and duration of the activity also contribute to the total heat stress. Since the body produces heat as it exercises, the higher
the intensity of the exercise and the longer the duration, the greater
will be the resulting heat load and the subsequent stress to the body.
It is possible to partially adapt or acclimatize to heat through repeated
exposure, but total adaptation never occurs, that is, it will always be
a major limitation to peak performance.

One of the primary concerns when exercising in the heat is dehydration. With high sweat rates, the body loses a large volume of water.
Since a major portion of this water loss comes from the blood volume,
a serious situation exists unless the individual rehydrates himself by
consuming the appropriate fluids. Water or a diluted electrolyte solution appear to be the best fluids for quick rehydration. Fluids high in
sugar content are not rapidly absorbed by the body. Since a salt loss
occurs with these high sweat rates, a liberal salting of food is recommended.

Since people respond quite differently to heat, the adjustments to
exercising in the heat should be made on an individual basis. In the
summer it is often important to exercise during the cooler parts of the
day, preferably when the sun's radiation is minimal (early morning or
early evening), to drink fluids abundantly, before, during, and following the exercise session, and to avoid exercise altogether when the
combination of temperature and humidity is such that severe heat stress
resulting in heat exhaustion or heat stroke is unavoidable. It is most
likely that both the intensity and duration of the activity will have to
be reduced to maintain the same training heart rate. In 1975, the American College of Sports Medicine published a position statement on,
"Prevention of Heat Injuries During Distance Running." This is included in Appendix B. Continued exposure to heat results in a gradual
adaptation (acclimatization) of the body to this stress, and the heat
can be tolerated much more effectively. If a participant must play
vigorous game activities or run races in the heat, then much of his or

her training should be done under similar conditions. For example, many runners had a bad experience at the 1975 Boston Marathon when the temperature soared over 90°F. They had not prepared themselves for the heat. One can become more than 90 percent acclimatized in approximately 14 days. If one becomes sporadic in exercising in the heat and chooses to train in the cool part of the day, then part of acclimatization is lost in just a few days.

COLD. Exercise in the cold presents far fewer problems. The exercise itself provides considerable body heat, and additional clothing can always be worn. Since the hands, feet, and head are particularly sensitive to extreme cold, proper gloves, extra socks, and a stocking hat with a face mask are strongly advised. As with heat, the degree of humidity and air movement are important. The more humid the air and the greater the wind velocity, the greater the cold stress for the same absolute temperature. On the other hand, in a very dry, cold environment, care must be taken not to overdress, since sweating will occur once the individual warms up and the sweat soaked clothing is subject to evaporation, which leads to rapid cooling and chills. If possible, easily unzipped layers of light clothing that can be ventilated (opened from the front), or even removed, are often better than one or two heavy garments. Table 7.1 outlines the interaction between temperature and wind speed and should be used as a guide to plan winter exercise sessions.

AIR POLLUTION. Air pollution has become a major consideration over the recent years because of its effect on the exercising subject. Although this may not be a problem in many rural communities, it is a major problem in most large metropolitan areas. Carbon monoxide has a much greater affinity or attraction to hemoglobin than oxygen. Since almost all oxygen is transported through the blood by hemoglobin, high concentrations of carbon monoxide greatly reduce one's working capacity. Other air pollutants have also been shown to have a significant effect on exercise capacity. In certain areas of the United States, smog alerts have been instituted to warn individuals to stay indoors and to restrict physicial activity levels on days when smog levels exceed a certain critical level. Exercising along heavily traveled roads can also expose the exerciser to fairly high, concentrated doses of pollutants, which are also potentially dangerous. Exercising in nonpolluted areas or restricting activity when pollution levels are high are both strongly suggested.

TABLE 7.1 Wind-Chill-Factor chart[a]

ESTIMATED WIND SPEED (mph)	ACTUAL THERMOMETER READING (°F)					
	50	40	30	20	10	0
	EQUIVALENT TEMPERATURE (°F)					
Calm	50	40	30	20	10	0
5	48	37	27	16	6	−5
10	40	28	16	4	−9	−24
15	36	22	9	−5	−18	−32
20	32	18	4	−10	−25	−39
25	30	16	0	−15	−29	−44
30	28	13	−2	−18	−33	−48
35	27	11	−4	−20	−35	−51
40	26	10	−6	−21	−37	−53
	Green				Yellow	
Wind speeds greater than 40 mph have little additional effect.)	LITTLE DANGER (for properly clothed person). Maximum danger of false sense of security.				INCREASING DANGER Danger from freezing or exposed flesh.	

Trenchfoot and immersion foot may occur at any point on this chart.

[a] Adapted from *Runner's World 8:* 28 (1973). Reproduced by permission of the publisher.

TABLE 7.1 (continued)

ACTUAL THERMOMETER READING (°F)

−10	−20	−30	−40	−50	−60

EQUIVALENT TEMPERATURE (°F)

−10	−20	−30	−40	−50	−60
−15	−26	−36	−47	−57	−68
−33	−46	−58	−70	−83	−95
−45	−58	−72	−85	−99	−112
−53	−67	−82	−96	−110	−124
−59	−74	−88	−104	−118	−133
−63	−79	−94	−109	−125	−140
−67	−82	−98	−113	−129	−145
−69	−85	−100	−116	−132	−148

Red

GREAT DANGER

ALTITUDE. The percentage of oxygen in the atmosphere at a 10,-000 foot altitude is exactly the same as that at sea level. However, the atmospheric pressure is much less at the 10,000 foot altitude, and thus pressure exerted by oxygen at that altitude is proportionally less than at sea level. As a result, it is more difficult to deliver oxygen to the working muscles of the body, and the absolute working capacity is reduced in direct proportion to the altitude. This will have little if any effect on short bursts of activity such as sprinting, but it will greatly affect activities of an endurance nature. For the same heart rate, more work can be done at sea level than at high altitude. As a result, the intensity of the workout at high altitudes should be reduced to maintain approximately the same cardiovascular stress as experienced at sea level. The body starts to adapt to the stress of a particular altitude shortly after arriving at that altitude. After several weeks at that altitude the body partially acclimatizes, but performance is still compromised.

AGE AND SEX CONSIDERATIONS

Do different individuals adapt differently to exercise, depending upon their age and sex? Are we "over the hill" by the age of 30 years? Are females genetically inferior to males when it comes to exercise capacity? These questions have been asked for many years and the answers are just now starting to surface.

First, endurance capacity does increase with age up to the middle to late twenties. Strength, muscular endurance, and cardiovascular endurance follow similar patterns of development. Females tend to reach their peak much earlier, that is, shortly after puberty. Males tend to maintain their peak values until the age of thirty, after which there is a gradual decline throughout their lives. Females start to decline shortly after attaining their peak and maintain a gradual decline throughout the rest of their lives. The earlier peak and decline for women is thought to be a result of their lack of participation at an early age. Up to the point of puberty, there are essentially no differences between males and females for practically all aspects of physical performance, that is, speed, strength, power, agility, muscular and cardiorespiratory endurance. Beyond puberty, the males become considerably stronger in upper body strength, faster, and have greater power, muscular and cardiorespiratory endurance.

Two trends emerge from the above that lead to the obvious questions: "Are the sex differences seen after puberty genetically determined, or are they the result of different cultural and social conditions, that is, the fact that women frequently discontinue participation in sports after puberty," and "Are the declines in physical ability noted with aging purely biological phenomena, or are they the result of an increasingly sedentary life-style?" To answer the first question, studies that have compared highly trained female athletes with male athletes of similar training have found few physiological differences between the sexes, with the exception of upper body strength. Therefore, it appears that the large differences seen between "normal" males and females beyond the age of puberty are the result of comparing moderately active males against relatively sedentary females. The implications are obvious. The female is not a second class citizen physically, but can enjoy all the same benefits of exercise enjoyed by the male!

With respect to the decline in performance with age, recent studies have shown that individuals who have remained physically active, even to the point of international class competition for their age category, have not experienced the same rate of decline in physiological function. There does appear to be a decrease, as would be expected, but the decrease is greatly accentuated by a decrease in daily physical activity patterns. Since there are a large number of men and women who are vigorously active in their 50s, 60s, and 70s (and even older), including those who are competing in 26-mile, 385-yard marathon runs, it does appear that age is not a barrier to an active life-style. For example, Dr. Fred Kasch, an adult fitness expert from San Diego, California, studied a group of middle-aged men who trained for 10 years (from age 45 to 55). The men maintained both their level of training and cardiorespiratory fitness. The older individual may need to start the exercise program at a much lower level and progress at a slower rate, but given time, the benefits will be the same.

SPECIFICITY OF TRAINING

Over the past few years, research has continued to confirm what many have suspected for years, that is, training benefits are specific to the activity. Athletes who participate in both football and basketball are frequently shocked to find that all of the hard training that conditioned them for the sport of football did little to prepare them for a full court scrimmage on the first night of basketball practice. Playing basketball conditions players for a game of basketball, but does little to prepare them for running a five mile race. Endurance training in a swimming pool has little or no carry over for long distance running. Changes that result from physical training are very specific to the actual muscles involved and to the pattern in which the muscles are used. This is an important concept to remember. Researchers are just now probing into why the training responses are so specific.

EXERCISE PROGRAMS FOR TRAVELING AND AT HOME

Frequently, an individual just gets started on an exercise program when the program is interrupted by a vacation, business travel, or inclement weather. This problem has been of major concern to physicians, exercise physiologists, and program staff, since this interruption frequently signals the end of the program for that particular individual. By the time he or she returns, or the weather improves, the urge and the desire to exercise has passed.

To combat the above situation, several different approaches have been taken to develop indoor home and travel programs in order to maintain the continuity of the exercise program. Some good indoor activities are available. The stationary bicycle is probably the best home exercise device. It can be set in front of the television or by an outside window to provide variety while exercising, thus eliminating potential boredom. Stationary bicycles should have an adjustable knob to vary the resistance against which the individual pedals. The resistance should be set to provide an intensity of exercise equivalent to that used in the individual's jogging, running, or swimming program, that is, use the same training heart rate. Duration and frequency would also be the same as that prescribed for jogging, walking, or swimming. Because of "specificity of training," it will probably take a few workouts to get the legs sufficiently in shape for a full program.

Rope skipping and running in place are two additional exercises that can be performed indoors at home, or when traveling on the road. Both exercises are excellent when performed correctly for the same duration and frequency, and at the same intensity as mentioned above for stationary cycling. A word of caution is necessary, however. Extreme muscle soreness in the calf muscles is very common during the first few weeks of both rope skipping and running in place programs. As with all other forms of exercise, the intensity is regulated on the basis of the training heart rate. Also, calf stretching exercises will help alleviate muscle soreness and cramping.

When traveling, it is also possible to substitute long, brisk walks, or stair climbing for the activity normally pursued. It is also becoming widely acceptable for joggers and runners to take their workout gear with them on trips. Usually there are parks or lightly traveled roads within a short distance of most hotels or motels. Once the individual overcomes the embarrassment of riding the elevator and walking through the lobby in his or her running gear, the rest is easy!

MOTIVATION

The success or failure of any exercise program is directly related to the motivation of the individual participants. Those who are highly motivated will continue their exercise program indefinitely, even when faced with injury. Those who are poorly motivated will have great difficulty adhering to their exercise program. It has been estimated that only 50 to 70 percent of those who start an exercise program will adhere to this program for 10 weeks or longer while the remaining 30 to 50 percent drop out. Studies have attempted to identify those factors that might be responsible for adherence versus dropout. Some of these include the attitude of the participant's husband or wife toward involvement in the program, the participant's credit rating, the proximity of the participant to the testing and exercise facility, the intensity of training, other commitments, and the freedom from serious illness or injury. Factors such as behavior pattern, health consciousness, attitude toward physical activity, level of physical fitness, previous athletic experiences, and social class apparently have little or no relationship to adherence rates. Factors that have not been studied, but would appear to be important, include the degree of supervison and guidance provided in the exercise program and the optimization of the exercise prescription, that is, mode, frequency, intensity, and duration.

Physical activity must be a life time pursuit, and therefore proper motivation is critical to continued participation in the exercise program. One of the most important aspects of motiviation is to have participants properly educated as to *why* regular exercise is an important component of their life-style. Films, books, bookets, lectures, seminars, workshops, or group discussions are all excellent methods to help them understand the importance of regular physical activity.

A second factor of equal importance is having participants engage in activities they enjoy, or helping them to learn to enjoy activities that would be of greatest benefit to them. Unfortunately, too many people have been under the false impression that jogging or running are the only activities that have any long-term benefit and value. Many people simply do not enjoy jogging or running. To insist that all people must jog or run is creating a situation where a high percentage of the participants will drop out of the exercise program after a relatively short period of time. Alternate activities that have a high aerobic or cardiorespiratory endurance component should be suggested and prescribed if they are more attractive to the participant. Brisk walking, hiking, swimming, bicycling, and vigorous sports such as handball, racquetball, and tennis would all be acceptable substitutes for jogging or running. While individuals may not improve as rapidly with these alternative modes of exercise, the important factor is that they will improve, and they have an entire lifetime ahead of them in which to attain optimal levels of fitness. It is argued by some, with good logic, that you should not use a sport to gain physical fitness but rather to maintain fitness through the sport. In other words, rather than using tennis as an activity to get into shape, use an activity like jogging for for several months to increase the basic level of fitness to a respectable level and then switch to tennis to maintain that optimal level. It is felt that the individual will be better able to enjoy participation in the sport if this approach is followed.

Other factors that have been shown to facilitate adherence include exercising at a regular time of day as a fixed part of a daily routine. Professionals who have conducted fitness programs for many years generally agree that the attrition rate is much lower for those who exercise in the early morning prior to going to work. First, there is the obvious advantage that there are few interruptions early in the morning—no phone calls, unscheduled meetings, early dinner, and so on. Second, when the weather is warm, this is an ideal time to exercise, since heat stress is minimized. However, it must be recognized that not everyone is a "morning person," and an early morning program would be largely unacceptable to some participants. Whatever the agreed upon time, consistency is the critical factor.

Exercising with a partner, or as a member of a formal group, as opposed to doing it alone, has been found to reduce the dropout rate.

Companionship and knowing that others are waiting is a potent motivator to show up for group exercise sessions. A word of caution must be introduced at this point, however. Group participation frequently leads to competition, and this is to be strongly discouraged. Almost everyone is intrigued by competition, but it is unwise for the novice who is just beginning his or her exercise program. Medical risks are involved as well as the potential for orthopedic and psychological injuries.

Simple tests, self-administered on a regular basis, are also motivating, as progress can be seen from week to week. Monitoring the resting pulse rate prior to getting up in the morning, following a good night's sleep, should show a decrease of approximately 1 beat per minute every two weeks for the first 15 to 20 weeks that the individual is in the exercise program. After 10 weeks in the program it is not unusual to see a resting pulse rate of 70 beats per minute drop to 65 beats per minute. This change reflects improvement in cardiorespiratory efficiency, which is a positive reinforcement to the participant and acts to encourage the individual to continue the present program. Many simple tests are available, can be self-administered, and certainly help to maintain a high level of participant enthusiasm and motivation.

The ultimate in motivation has been recently noted by Dr. William Glasser, who in his book, *Positive Addiction*, has reported that joggers or runners who exercise 30 to 60 minutes per day, four days per week or more, frequently become addicted to this routine. If illness, injury, travel, or some other interruption disrupts their exercise routine, these individuals actually go through withdrawal like symptoms. Of course, this would be a highly desirable outcome, but unfortunately too many individuals do not have the patience, persistence, or psychological strength to get to this point of "positive addiction."

Most recently, attempts have been made to apply the concepts of behavioral modification to increase adherence to exercise programs. Since this is a new approach, it is too early to predict if it will be any more successful than traditional approaches. Behavior modification uses a system of rewards for changes in behavior. Many programs have been providing rewards to their participants in the form of 100 Mile Club, 500 Mile Club, 1,000 Mile Club and 10,000 Mile Club T-shirts. These programs have been shown to be very effective. It is somewhat ironic to watch mature men, who are wealthy enough to buy the entire company that makes the T-shirts, fight to get one of these relatively inexpensive rewards. If past experience provides any indication of the future, behavior modification techniques, applied more broadly, should have a significant impact on increasing adherence rates.

SUMMARY

Participation in any exercise program requires that attention be given to a number of factors, each of which directly influences how successful the individual participant will be in his or her exercise program. Ignoring such things as correct shoes, clothing, and special equipment; warm-up, cool-down, and injury prevention; and environmental factors such as heat, cold, humidity, air pollution, and altitude can lead the participant into an unpleasant if not hazardous situation that may have tragic consequences. A knowledge of the specificity of training and how the sexes and individuals of varying ages differ in their response to an exercise program is also extremely important. Total education of the participant is important to prevent possible medical complications or injury, and to promote a healthy, positive attitude toward the program. Exercise must become the reward, and not the punishment.

REFERENCES

1. Åstrand, I. "Aerobic work capacity—its relation to age, sex, and other factors." *Circ. Res.*, Supplement I, Vols, 20 and 21, *I*: 211-217 (1967).

2. Barnard, R.J., G.W. Gardner, N.V. Diaco, R.N. MacAlpin, and A.A. Kattus. "Cardiovascular responses to sudden strenuous exercise—heart rate, blood pressure, and ECG." *J. Appl. Physiol.*, *34*:833-834 (1973).

3. Bottiger, L.E. "Regular decline in physical working capacity with age." *Brit. Med. J.*, *3*:270-271 (1973).

4. Buskirk, E., and D. Bas. "Climate and exercise." In: *Science and Medicine on Exercise and Sports*, W.R. Johnson (ed.). New York: Harper and Brothers, 1960, pp. 311-338.

5. Cureton, T.K. "A physical fitness case study of Joie Ray (Improving physical fitness from age 60 to 70 years)." *J. Ass. Phys. Mental Rehab.*, *18*:64-72 (1964).

6. Drinkwater, B.L., P.B. Raven, S.M. Horvath, J.A. Gliner, R.O. Ruhling, N.W. Bolduan, and S. Taguchi. "Air pollution, ex-

ercise, and heat stress." *Arch. Environ. Health, 28*:177-181 (1974).

7. Glasser, W. *Positive Addiction.* New York: Harper and Row. 1976.

8. Gliner, J.A., P.B. Raven, S.M. Horvath, B.L. Drinkwater, and J.C. Sutton. "Man's physiologic response to long-term work during thermal and pollutant stress." *J. Appl. Physiol., 39*:628-632 (1975).

9. Goddard, R.F. (ed.). *The Effects of Altitude on Physical Performance.* Chicago: The Athletic Institute, 1966.

10. Grimby, G., and B. Saltin, "Physiological analysis of physically well-trained middle-aged and old athletes." *Acta Med. Scand., 179:*513-526 (1966).

11. Horvath. S.M., P.B. Raven, T.E. Dahms, and D.J. Gray. "Maximal aerobic capacity at different levels of carboxyhemoglobin." *J. Appl. Physiol., 38*:300-303 (1975).

12. Morgan W.P. "Involvement in vigorous physical activity with special reference to adherence." Proceedings: National College of Physical Education for Men, Orlando, Fla., Jan 1977.

13. Murphy, R., and W. Ashe. "Prevention of heat illness in football players." JAMA, *194*:650-654 (1965).

14. Pollock, M.L., G.A. Dawson, H.S. Miller, Jr., A. Ward, D. Cooper, W. Headley, A.C. Linnerud, and M.M. Nomeir. "Physiologic responses of men 49 to 65 years of age to endurance training." *J. Amer. Geriat. Soc., 24*:97-104 (1976).

15. Pollock, M.L., L.R. Gettman, C.A. Milesis, M.D. Bah, L. Durstine, and R.B. Johnson. "Effects of frequency and duration of training on attrition and incidence of injury." *Med. Sci. Sports. 9*:31-36 (1977).

16. Raven, P.B., B.L. Drinkwater, R.O. Ruhling, N.W. Bolduan, S. Taguchi, J.A. Gliner, and S.M. Horvath. "Effect of carbon monoxide and peroxyacetylinitrate on man's maximal aerobic capacity." *J. Appl. Physiol., 36*:228-293 (1974).

17. Raven, P.B., B.L. Drinkwater, S.M. Horvath, J.A. Gliner, R.O. Ruhling, J.C. Sutton, and N.W. Bolduan. "Age, smoking habits, heat stress, and their interactive effects with carbon monoxide and peroxyacetylnitrate on man's aerobic power." *Inter. J. Bio-*

meteorol., *18*:222-232 (1974).

18. Roby, F.G., and R.P. Davis. *Jogging for Fitness and Weight Control.* Philadelphia: W.B. Saunders, 1970.

19. Sharkey, B.J. *Fitness and Work Capacity.* U.S. Department of Agriculture, Forest Service Equipment Development Center, Missoula, Montana, 1976.

20. Skinner, J.S. "Age and performance." In: *Limiting Factors of Physical Performance.* Stuttgart: George Thieme Publishers, 1973, pp. 271-282.

21. Wilmore, J.H., H.S. Miller, and M.L. Pollock. "Body composition and physiological characteristics of active endurance athletes in their eighth decade of life." *Med. Sci. Sports, 6*:44-48 (1974).

22. Wilmore J.H. "Inferiority of female athletes: myth or reality." *J. Sports Med., 3*:1-6 (1975).

23. Zohman, L.R. *Beyond diet. . . exercise your way to fitness and heart health.* Englewood Cliffs, N.J.: Mazola Products, Best Foods, 1974.

Appendix A
Evaluation Procedures, Norms and Data Forms

CARDIORESPIRATORY FITNESS

The purpose of this section is to provide additional detailed information concerning the medical and fitness evaluation procedures. Table A.1 shows an example of an informed consent form and Table A.2, a medical history form. Remember though, forms should be individualized for the local situation.

EMERGENCY PROCEDURES. The knowledge of emergency procedures is essential when conducting fitness evaluations and exercise programs. All personnel involved with the program must be informed of such procedures, trained in cardiopulmonary resuscitation and basic first aid, and be able to determine the severity of the emergency and make the appropriate response. All personnel should have assigned duties in an emergency and should practice these duties regularly to ensure teamwork and reduce possible confusion that may occur during an actual emergency. The procedures for action during an emergency should be typed and posted, and should be continually updated. The most recent information concerning cardiopulmonary resuscitation and first aid procedures should be reviewed frequently with the staff (three months interim is recommended). The equipment on hand for emergencies should include the items listed in Table A.3. A telephone code system is recommended to expedite communication with the referring physician or hospital.

TABLE A.1. Informed consent for exercise testing*

Institute for Aerobics Research
11811 Preston Road
Dallas, Texas 75230

The undersigned hereby voluntarily consents to engage in a maximum exercise test to determine the maximum oxygen intake and cardiovascular function. The test will be monitored continuously by an electrocardiogram recording and oscilloscope. This test will facilitate evaluation of cardiopulmonary function and assist the physician or exercise physiologist in prescribing or evaluating exercise programs. It is my understanding that I will be questioned and examined by a physician prior to taking the test and will be given a resting electrocardiogram to exclude contraindications to such testing.

Exercise testing will be performed by running, walking, swimming or riding a bicycle, with the workload increasing every few minutes until fatigue or breathlessness or other symptoms dictate cessation of the test. Blood pressure and electrocardiogram will be monitored by a physician or trained exercise physiologist. In the latter case, a physician will be readily available in case of emergency.

There exists the possibility that certain changes may occur during the progress of the test. These changes could include abnormal heart beats, abnormal blood pressure and in rare instances a "heart attack". Professional care in selection and supervision of individuduals provides appropriate precaution against such problems.

The benefits of such testing are the scientific assessment of working capacity and the clinical appraisal of health hazards which will facilitate prescription of conditioning-rehabilitative exercise. Records will be held in strict confidence from non-medical people (such as employers and insurance agents) unless consent is obtained. The welfare of persons being tested is safeguarded by professional care and by the availability of emergency treatment should it be necessary.

Finally, I permit registration of my name for possible follow-up purposes in the future.

Further, the undersigned releases and discharges the Institute for Aerobics Research, its officers, agents, staff, faculty, physicians, technicians and any others connected therewith from all claims or damages whatsoever that the undersigned or his representative may have arising from, or incident to this test.

Signed _____

Witness _____

Date _____

Physician or Exercise Physiologist Supervising Test

*Published with permission of the Institute for Aerobics Research, Dallas, Texas.

TABLE A.2. Medical history questionnaire*

TABLE A-2

MEDICAL HISTORY QUESTIONNAIRE

Institute for Aerobics Research
11811 Preston Road
Dallas, Texas 75230

This is your medical history form for your visit to The Institute for Aerobics Research. All information will be kept confidentail. The doctor or exercise physiologist you see at the Institute will use this information in his evaluation of your health. You will want to make it as accurate and complete as possible, yet free of meaningless details. Please fill out this form carefully and thoroughly. Then check it over to be sure you haven't left out anything.

Note: Please **print** all responses so that your data will be compatible with computer storage and analysis.

Name _____ Exam Date _____ ,19 _____

*Published with permission of the Institute for Aerobics Research, Dallas, Texas.

TABLE A.2. (Continued) Medical history questionnaire

Institute for Aerobics Research
11811 Preston Road
Dallas, Texas 75230

Patient Medical History Form

All information is private and confidential. Please Print.

DO NOT WRITE IN THIS SPACE; FOR OFFICE USE ONLY.

PATIENT NUMBER	VISIT	CARD	FORM	CLINIC
		0 1	M 0 2	B

I. GENERAL INFORMATION

☐ Mr. NAME
☐ Ms.
☐ Miss FIRST   MIDDLE   LAST
☐ Mrs.
☐ Dr.

ADDRESS

NUMBER AND STREET

02 CITY   STATE ZIP CODE

COUNTRY (IF OUTSIDE U.S.A.)

HOME PHONE   SOCIAL SECURITY NUMBER   DATE OF BIRTH   TODAY'S DATE
( )   -   -   -   MONTH DAY YEAR   MONTH DAY YEAR
AREA CODE

FAMILY PHYSICIAN

Dr.
FIRST NAME, IF KNOWN   INITIAL LAST NAME

DOCTOR'S ADDRESS (if known)

NUMBER AND STREET   PHONE

04 CITY   STATE ZIP CODE   AREA CODE ( )   -

May we send a copy of your consult to your physician?   Yes ☐   No ☐

MARITAL STATUS

Single ☐   Married ☐   Divorced ☐   Widowed ☐   Separated ☐

SEX

Male ☐   Female ☐   PRESENT AGE

EDUCATION (Check highest level attained)

☐ Grade School   ☐ High School   ☐ College Graduate

☐ Junior High School   ☐ Two-year College (or 4-year college;   ☐ Postgraduate School
                            degree not completed)

OCCUPATION

FOR OFFICE USE ONLY

OCCUP CODE ☐

EMPLOYER (use abbreviations if necessary)

05

EMPLOYER'S ADDRESS

NUMBER AND STREET   BUSINESS PHONE

06 CITY   STATE ZIP CODE   AREA CODE ( )   -

What is/are your purpose(s) in coming to the Institute?

☐ To participate in a research study.

☐ To determine my current level of physical fitness and to receive recommendations for an exercise program.

☐ Other (please explain):

07

PLEASE PRINT

TABLE A.2. (Continued) Medical history questionnaire

When dates are required, please use numbers to represent the months as follows:

January 01	May 05	September 09
February 02	June 06	October 10
March 03	July 07	November 11
April 04	August 08	December 12

For addresses, please use the official Post Office two-letter abbreviations listed below.

Abbreviations for States (and Territories)

AL	Alabama		NE	Nebraska
AK	Alaska		NV	Nevada
AZ	Arizona		NH	New Hampshire
AR	Arkansas		NJ	New Jersey
CA	California		NM	New Mexico
CZ	Canal Zone (Panama)		NY	New York
CO	Colorado		NC	North Carolina
CT	Connecticut		ND	North Dakota
DE	Delaware		OH	Ohio
FL	Florida		OK	Oklahoma
GA	Georgia		OR	Oregon
GU	Guam		PA	Pennsylvania
HI	Hawaii		PR	Puerto Rico
ID	Idaho		RI	Rhode Island
IL	Illinois		SC	South Carolina
IN	Indiana		SD	South Dakota
IA	Iowa		TN	Tennessee
KS	Kansas		TX	Texas
KY	Kentucky		UT	Utah
LA	Louisiana		VT	Vermont
ME	Maine		VA	Virginia
MD	Maryland		VI	Virgin Islands
MA	Massachusetts		WA	Washington (state)
MI	Michigan		DC	Washington, D. C.
MN	Minnesota		WV	West Virginia
MS	Mississippi		WI	Wisconsin
MO	Missouri		WY	Wyoming
MT	Montana			

TABLE A.2. (Continued) Medical history questionnaire

Medical History

PATIENT NUMBER	VISIT	CARD	FORM	CLINIC	2
		1	0	M	0	2	8

PRESENT HISTORY

Check the box in front of those questions to which your answer is yes. Leave others blank.

10

Has a doctor ever said that your blood pressure was too high or too low?
Do you ever have pain in your heart or chest?
Are you often bothered by a thumping of the heart?
Does your heart often race like mad?
Do you ever notice extra heart beats or skipped beats?
Are your ankles often badly swollen?
Do cold hands or feet trouble you even in hot weather?
Has a doctor ever said that you had or have heart trouble,
an abnormal electrocardiogram (ECG or EKG), heart attack, or coronary?
Do you suffer from frequent cramps in your legs?
Do you often have difficulty breathing?
Do you get out of breath long before anyone else?
Do you sometimes get out of breath when sitting still or sleeping?
Has a doctor ever told you your cholesterol level was high?

Comments:

11

12

13

Do you now have or have you recently had:

14

A chronic, recurrent or morning cough?
Any episode of coughing up blood?
Increased anxiety or depression?
Problems with recurrent fatigue, trouble sleeping or increased
irritability?
Migraine or recurrent headaches?
Swollen or painful knees or ankles?
Swollen, stiff or painful joints?
Pain in your legs after walking short distances?
Back pain?
Kidney problems such as passing stones, burning, increased frequency,
decreased force of stream of difficulty in starting or stopping your stream?
Prostate trouble (men only)?
Any stomach or intestinal problems such as recurrent heartburn,
ulcers, constipation or diarrhea?
Any significant vision or hearing problem?
Any recent change in a wart or mole?
Glaucoma or increased pressure in the eyes?
Exposure to loud noises for long periods?

Comments:

15

WOMEN ONLY answer the following:

16

Do you have any menstrual period problems?
Do you have problems with recurrent itching or discharge?
Did you have any significant childbirth problems?
Do you have any breast discharges or lumps?
Do you sometimes lose urine when you cough, sneeze or laugh?

Please give number of: Pregnancies |___|___| Living children |___| First day of last |___|___|___| menstrual period MONTH DAY YEAR

Date of last pelvic exam and/or Paps smear: month |___| year 19 |___| Results: Normal |___| Abnormal |___|

Comments:

17

PLEASE PRINT

TABLE A.2. (Continued) Medical history questionnaire

Medical History

MEN and WOMEN answer the following:

DO NOT WRITE IN THIS SPACE; FOR OFFICE USE ONLY.

PATIENT NUMBER	VISIT	CARD	FORM	CLINIC
		2 5	M 0 2	B

3

List any prescribed medications you are now taking:

[25]

List any self-prescribed medications or dietary supplements you are now taking:

[26]

Date of last complete physical examination: _____ month 19 _____ year never ☐ can't remember ☐ Normal ☐ Abnormal ☐

[27]

Date of last chest x-ray: _____ month 19 _____ year never ☐ can't remember ☐ Normal ☐ Abnormal ☐

Date of last electrocardiogram: _____ month 19 _____ year never ☐ can't remember ☐ Normal ☐ Abnormal ☐

Date of last dental check-up: _____ month 19 _____ year never ☐ can't remember ☐ Normal ☐ Abnormal ☐

List any other medical or diagnostic test you have had in the past two years:

[28]

[29]

List hospitalizations including dates of and reasons for hospitalization:

[30]

[31]

[32]

List any drug allergies:

[33]

PAST HISTORY

Have you ever had:

[34]

☐ Heart Attack, how many years ago? _____
☐ Rheumatic Fever
☐ Heart murmur
☐ Diseases of the arteries
☐ Varicose veins
☐ Arthritis of legs or arms
☐ Diabetes or abnormal blood sugar test
☐ Phlebitis
☐ Dizziness or fainting spells
☐ Epilepsy or fits
☐ Strokes
☐ Diphtheria
☐ Scarlet fever
☐ Infectious mononucleosis
☐ Anemia

☐ Thyroid problems
☐ Pneumonia
☐ Bronchitis
☐ Asthma
☐ Abnormal chest x-ray
☐ Other lung diseases
☐ Injuries to back, arms, legs or joints
☐ Broken bones
☐ Jaundice or gallbladder problems
☐ Polio
☐ Urinary tract infections, kidney stones, or prostate problems.
☐ Any nervous or emotional problems

Comments:

[35]

PLEASE PRINT

TABLE A.2. (Continued) Medical history questionnaire

Medical History

FAMILY MEDICAL HISTORY

40 FATHER: Alive ☐   Current age ☐ │ General health now: excellent ☐₁ good ☐₂ fair ☐₃ poor ☐₄ don't know ☐₅
Deceased ☐   Age at death ☐ │ Cause of death or reason for poor health now: ☐

MOTHER: Alive ☐   Current age ☐ │ General health now: excellent ☐₁ good ☐₂ fair ☐₃ poor ☐₄ don't know ☐₅
Deceased ☐   Age at death ☐ │ Cause of death or reason for poor health now: ☐

41 SIBLINGS: No. of brothers ☐   No. of sisters ☐   Age range ☐ – ☐   Health Problems: ☐

FAMILIAL DISEASES: Have any of your blood relatives had any of the following?
Include grandparents, aunts, and uncles, but exclude cousins, relatives by marriage, and half relatives.

42
☐ Heart attacks under age 50
☐ Strokes under age 50
☐ High blood pressure
☐ Elevated cholesterol
☐ Diabetes
☐ Asthma or hay fever

☐ Congenital heart disease
☐ Heart operations
☐ Glaucoma
☐ Obesity (20 or more lbs. overweight)
☐ Leukemia or cancer under age 60

Comments: ☐

43

OTHER HEART DISEASES RISK FACTORS

44 SMOKING

Have you ever smoked cigarettes, cigars or a pipe?   yes ☐₁   no ☐₂
If no, skip to Diet section.
Do you smoke presently?   yes ☐   no ☐
If you did or do smoke cigarettes, how many per day? ☐   Age you started: ☐
If you did or do smoke cigars, how many per day? ☐   Age you started: ☐
If you did or do smoke a pipe, how many pipefuls per day? ☐   Age you started: ☐
If you have quit smoking, when was it? ☐ MONTH 19 ☐ YEAR

45 DIET

What do you consider a good weight for yourself? ☐ pounds

What is the most you have ever weighed? (including when pregnant) ☐ lbs.   At what age? ☐ yrs.

Weight: Now ☐ lbs.   One year ago ☐ lbs.   At age 21 ☐ lbs.

Number of meals you usually eat per day. ☐

Average number of eggs you usually eat per week: ☐   (Do not count those in cooking and baking, cakes, casseroles, etc.)

Number of times per week you usually eat:

Beef ☐   Fish ☐   Desserts ☐
Pork ☐   Fowl ☐   French fried foods ☐

Number of servings (cups, glasses or containers) per week you usually consume of:

Homogenized (whole) milk ☐   Buttermilk ☐
Skim (non-fat) milk ☐   Tea (iced or hot) ☐
Two percent (2% fat) milk ☐   Coffee ☐

Do you ever drink alcoholic beverages?   yes ☐   no ☐

If yes, what is your approximate intake of these beverages?

	None	Occasional	Often	If often, how many drinks per week?
Beer	☐	☐	☐	☐
Wine	☐	☐	☐	☐
Hard Liquor	☐	☐	☐	☐

At any time in the past were you a heavy drinker (consumption of 6 oz. of hard liquor per day or more)?   yes ☐₁   no ☐₂

46 Comments: ☐

PLEASE PRINT

TABLE A.2. (Continued) Medical history questionnaire

Medical History

EXERCISE

50 Are you currently involved in a regular exercise program?   yes ☐   no ☐

Do you regularly walk or run one or more miles continuously?   yes ☐   no ☐   don't know ☐

If yes, average no. of miles you cover per workout or day: ☐ . ☐ miles

What is your average time per mile? ☐ : ☐ minutes: seconds   don't know ☐

Do you practice weight lifting or home calisthenics?   yes ☐   no ☐

Are you now involved in the Aerobics program?   yes ☐   no ☐

If yes, your average Aerobics points per week: ☐

Have you taken in the past 6 months: ☐ 12 minute test   ☐ 1.5 mile   ☐ neither

If yes, your miles in 12 minutes: ☐ . ☐   or your time for 1.5 miles: ☐ : ☐ minutes : seconds

Do you frequently participate in competitive sports?   yes ☐   no ☐

If yes, which one or ones?

☐ Golf   ☐ Bowling   ☐ Tennis   ☐ Handball   ☐ Soccer

☐ Basketball   ☐ Volleyball   ☐ Football   ☐ Baseball   ☐ Track

☐ Other _____

Average number of times per month ☐

51 In which of the following high school or college athletics did you participate?

☐ None   ☐ Football   ☐ Basketball   ☐ Baseball   ☐ Soccer

☐ Track   ☐ Swimming   ☐ Tennis   ☐ Wrestling   ☐ Golf

☐ Other _____

In which of the following high school or college athletics did you earn a varsity letter?

☐ None   ☐ Football   ☐ Basketball   ☐ Baseball   ☐ Soccer

☐ Track   ☐ Swimming   ☐ Tennis   ☐ Wrestling   ☐ Golf

☐ Other _____

52 What activity or activities would you prefer in a regular exercise program for yourself?

☐ Walking and/or running   ☐ Bicycling (outdoors)   ☐ Swimming

☐ Stationary running   ☐ Stationary cycling   ☐ Tennis

☐ Jumping rope   ☐ Handball, basketball or squash

☐ Other _____

53 Comments: _____

Explain any other significant medical problems that you consider important for us to know:

5 5 _____

5 6 _____

5 7 _____

5 8 _____

5 9 _____

6 0 _____

6 1 _____

PLEASE PRINT

TABLE A.3. Emergency equipment and drugs needed for testing and training locations.

EQUIPMENT	DRUGS
1. Defibrillator (portable synchronized DC preferable)	1. Morphine or meperidine
2. Oxygenator, intermittent positive-pressure capability	2. Nitroglycerin tablets and amyl nitrite pearls
3. Airways, oral and endotracheal	3. Catecholamines Aramine Epinephrine 1/10,000 IV Norepinephrine IV Isoproterenol IV
4. Bag-valve-mask hand respirator (Hope nonrebreathing bag)	4. Antiarrhythmics Lidocaine IV Procainamide IV Propranolol IV/oral
5. Syringes and needles	5. Atropine sulfate
6. Intravenous sets	6. Digoxin, cedilanid-lanatoside C
7. Intravenous stand	7. Sodium bicarbonate solution
8. Adhesive tape	8. Dextrose, 5% in water
9. Laryngoscope (desirable)	9. Lasix (furosemide) IV
10. First-aid kit	10. Tensilon (edrophonium)

With respect to the use of equipment listed in Table A.3, the non-physician should not start an IV, or administer drugs to an individual (unless advised to do so by a physician), but should mainly be involved in basic cardiopulmonary resuscitation procedures. Because most persons who collapse during exercise do so from a ventricular dysrhythmia, the indications for and use of a defibrillator is imperative for paramedical (allied health) personnel. Local laws and customs vary as to what nonphysicians should or are allowed to do.

Some cardiac rehabilitation and adult fitness programs have gone to a direct line call system to a local physician's office or hospital. The EGG system is connected to a telephone jack or CB radio, and therefore, by dialing a specific number, ECG records are sent directly to the physician's monitoring system. In this way, if an emergency occurs, trained paramedical personnel can be in direct contact with a physician immediately for diagnosis and emergency care. Although the initial cost for the interfacing of this equipment is expensive, it may be cheaper over the long haul if having a physician present is not feasable. Because of the difficulty in getting physician coverage at all times or its impracticality, many programs are shifting to this approach.

In regard to the participant, one should generally exercise where other persons are present. This would be particularly true with high-risk individuals because, in case of an emergency, someone would be available to get help and administer first aid.

SPECIAL CONSIDERATIONS IN THE SELECTION OF TESTS AND PERSONNEL. Often, the type of test battery administered to participants depends on four major factors: time, expense, qualifications of personnel, and the population to be tested. If large numbers of individuals have to be tested in a short time, the test items may be limited to a less sophisticated test battery. If high-risk persons are involved, the exercise tolerance test with ECG and blood pressure monitoring should always be used.

With persons over 35 years of age or high-risk individuals, a physician should be present during exercise testing. For this same group, field tests for determination of cardiorespiratory fitness, such as a one-mile to two-mile run, should not be attempted. The field tests would only be acceptable for use with young persons or middle-aged individuals who have been carefully screened and have had recent experience in jogging or running. A more definitive statement concerning subject safety has been established by the American Heart Association's committee on exercise. It states:

> *Emergency equipment and qualified personnel should be available for exercise testing of all persons. Patients with known or suspected heart disease or dysfunction should not be tested without a qualified physician at the site or in the immediate area (within 30 seconds) in order to provide life saving emergency care. In the case of younger individuals (under age 35), free of clinical abnormalities or increased risk factors, the untoward responses to exercise are extremely uncommon. Direct physician presence is not considered necessary provided the health care personnel directing the sessions are trained to the satisfaction of the responsible physician in cardiopulmonary resuscitation (CPR) and emergency cardiac care (ECC) according to standards set by the American Heart Association and the Committee on Emergency Medical Services of the National Academy of Sciences–National Research Council, Division of Medical Sciences.*

The expense of equipment often dictates the kind of equipment that will be available for testing. If funds are limited, the two most important pieces of equipment for exercise tolerance testing (cardiorespiratory fitness) would be an ECG recorder and blood pressure apparatus. Next, an oscilloscope and possibly a cardiotachometer could be purchased, followed by an exercise bicycle ergometer or treadmill. The oscilloscope would allow the tester to observe the ECG wave at all times, and the cardiotachometer provides an instant visual readout of heart rate.

It is understood from Section 2 that maximum oxygen uptake is one of the best measures of assessing cardiorespiratory fitness. If so, why haven't we said anything about the purchase of equipment to be used for this test? Maximum oxygen uptake can be estimated accurately from performance time on a treadmill, bicycle ergometer, or field tests (running); thus the need for actual measurement may not be necessary. Gas analyzers, a flow meter, and the extra personnel needed to assess the actual measure are not worth the added expense. Except for research purposes, a precise measurement is not necessary.

Having the right personnel available for the various phases of a physical fitness program is necessary. Although the physician and the program director have overall control of the program, they must have qualified exercise leaders and laboratory technicians to help them conduct the program. Exercise leaders should have a background in functional anatomy, exercise physiology, behavioral psychology and group dynamics, emergency procedures, and exercise prescription. The laboratory technician should have expertise in the mechanics of individual test procedures, screening a participant before exercise testing, administration of tests, and data analysis. Programs for training and certifying program directors, exercise leaders, and laboratory technicians are now available through the auspices of the American College of Sports Medicine.

TESTS AND PROCEDURES.   As listed in Table 3.2, there are a variety of tests available to determine cardiorespiratory fitness. They are generally classified as resting, submaximal, and maximal tests.

RESTING EVALUATION

The resting evaluation should include the determination of resting heart rate, blood pressure, and a 12-lead ECG. Standards for heart rate and blood pressure, subdivided by age and sex, are shown in Tables A.4 to A.13. The standard equipment used for the measurement of these parameters would include a stethoscope, stopwatch, sphygmomanometer (blood pressure cuff apparatus), and ECG recorder. A comfortable armchair should be used for determining heart rate and blood pressure and a stretcher bed or table for the resting ECG. For more information on resting and exercise ECGs, see references by Blackburn and Ellestad.

For persons who have a family history of valvular heart disease, are over 35 years of age, or are at a high risk for coronary heart disease, a physician should listen for specific heart and blood vessel abnormalities (auscultation). This is done by the physician's holding a stethoscope to various parts of the chest, back, neck, and elsewhere to listen to the heart beat, the sound of the valves of the heart opening and closing, and blood rushing through the vessels. This should be considered as part of a physical examination, since dangerous valve or vessel dysfunctions are found in this way. Some subtle sounds are of considerable importance to the clearance for an exercise program of high intensity.

The heart rate is usually counted for 15 or 30 seconds and then multiplied appropriately to get beats per minute. Blood pressure should be measured two to three times with the average value of both systolic and diastolic pressure being recorded. For best results in taking blood pressure:

1. Take the measurement in a quiet room with the temperature approximately 72°F.

2. Have the men with shirt already off and women dressed in a sleeveless blouse (this makes it easier to adjust the pressure cuff properly).

3. Take the blood pressure from both the left and right arms (because of arterial obstructions, sometimes the pressure in one arm is different from the other).

4. Use the proper size cuff (a large cuff on a small arm will cause the readings to be lower).

5. Take the measure fairly rapidly and leave the pressure cuff deflated for approximately 10 seconds between determinations (this will allow normal circulation to return to the arm).

In taking blood pressure, pump the gauge rapidly up to 180 to 200 millimeters of mercury, and ease it down fairly fast to within 20 millimeters of mercury of a person's estimated systolic blood pressure. Then slowly let out pressure until the first sound is heard. The first sound one hears in the stethoscope is the systolic pressure. This is the highest pressure in the artery and represents the pressure caused by the contraction of the heart muscle. The first pulse sound is followed by a series of different tones and, at a lower level, there is a change to a low muffled sound before disappearing. The low, muffled sound is called fourth phase diastolic pressure and the fifth phase is when the sound disappears. Usually just the fifth phase diastolic pressure is recorded at rest. Diastolic pressure represents the pressure in the artery when the heart is at rest. During recovery from exercise, the fifth phase diastolic blood pressure is often heard all the way to zero; thus both fourth and fifth phase should be noted.

Persons with a resting systolic blood pressure above 180 millimeters of mercury or diastolic blood pressure over 100 millimeters of mercury should be referred to a physician before further testing or training. In most cases it would be wiser to have a person reduce their blood pressure (drugs and/or a dietary control program) before letting them begin a training program. If someone is hypertensive, make sure the initial program is of a low intensity. The hypertensive person should also avoid moderate to heavy lifting or pushing exercises. These types of exercises have a dramatic effect on elevating the blood pressure.

EXERCISE TOLERANCE TESTING: THE DETERMINATION AND PREDICTION OF MAXIMUM AEROBIC CAPACITY

A critical concern regarding the evaluation of cardiorespiratory function evolves around the question: How strenuous should a test be? Many testers feel that a maximal or near maximal effort is necessary in most cases, while others favor a less strenuous evaluation. Taylor, Ellestad, and Wilson provide excellent reviews on procedures and concepts of stress testing for the diagnosis of coronary heart disease (CHD) and estimation of cardiorespiratory function (see reference numbers 17, 35, and 37 at the end of Section 3). Also, standards for maximum oxygen uptake can be found in Tables A.4 to A.13.

Theoretically, it would be advantageous to be able to stress test all participants at an intensity above which they will be training. Maximum stress testing is particularly recommended for athletic or occupational groups involved in near or maximal efforts. This would help to insure that the participant was adapting well physiologically to the training regimen. For example, several years ago, we had the opportunity to evaluate 33 Masters runners.* They averaged 47.4 years of age, were without symptoms of disease, and had been in training for over five years. All were administered a maximal treadmill stress test. The tests showed ECG evidence of severe disease in two men. One of these men had an enlarged heart resulting from valvular disease, had a dangerous rhythm disturbance, and demonstrated evidence of inadequate blood supply to the heart during exercise (called ischemia and is shown as ST segment depression on the ECG of more than 1 millimeter). See Figure A.1 for diagram of normal ECG tracing, one with ST segment depression, and one showing a premature ventricular beat. The unsettling fact here was that the competitor had not had a physical examination in a number of years and thought he was perfectly healthy. Subsequently, the person consulted a physician who took him off of the competitive running program. He continued to exercise, but at a much lower level of intensity.

*Persons competing in track competition who are 40 years of age and older.

TABLE A.4 Physical fitness and health standards for men 20 to 29 years of age[a]

PERCENTILE RANKINGS		RESTING (SITTING)			MAXIMUM
		HEART RATE (beats/min)	BLOOD PRESSURE SYSTOLIC (mmHg)	DIASTOLIC (mmHg)	OXYGEN UPTAKE (ml/kg·min)
High	99	40	94	60	60.0
	95	46	102	64	51.5
	90	50	110	70	47.5
Above average	85	52	110	70	46.5
	80	54	112	72	45.0
	75	56	116	75	43.8
	70	58	118	78	43.8
Average	65	59	120	78	42.5
	60	60	120	80	41.8
	55	62	120	80	41.0
	50	63	121	80	39.1
	40	66	128	80	37.0
	35	68	130	82	36.3
Below average	30	70	130	84	35.6
	25	71	132	85	35.5
	20	72	136	88	33.5
	15	76	140	90	32.5
Low	10	80	140	90	31.5
	5	88	150	100	29.0
	1	99	158	110	22.8
Population size		358	367	367	371
Average		64	124	80	40.0
Standard deviation		12.5	13.4	9.6	6.4

[a]Data comes from the Cooper Clinic Coronary Risk Factor Profile Charts which are from data collected on patients being evaluated at the Cooper Clinic and standards being established at the Institute for Aerobics Research, Dallas, Texas. Published with permission.

TABLE A.4. (Continued) Physical fitness and health standards for men 20 to 29 years of age

MAXIMUM				
HEART RATE (beats/min)	CHOLES-TEROL (mg%)	TRIGLY-CERIDES (mg%)	GLUCOSE (mg%)	FAT (%)
214	120	27	75	7.2
209	142	48	83	9.6
205	154	55	88	11.6
202	160	62	90	12.9
200	165	66	93	13.9
200	172	71	95	15.3
199	178	76	96	16.2
198	185	82	98	17.1
197	190	87	100	18.0
196	195	93	100	19.1
194	199	100	102	20.1
192	203	110	103	21.2
191	207	123	104	22.3
190	211	137	105	23.4
188	218	148	105	25.4
186	222	170	106	27.4
183	229	180	109	28.6
180	240	200	110	30.5
179	251	234	113	32.8
170	269	296	118	38.0
145	300	762	123	49.0
371	273	271	271	248
192	200	133	101	21.6
12.2	39.1	107.8	14.5	9.1

TABLE A.5. Physical fitness and health standards for men 30 to 39 years of age[a]

PERCENTILE RANKINGS		RESTING (SITTING)			MAXIMUM
		HEART RATE (beats/min)	BLOOD PRESSURE SYSTOLIC (mmHg)	DIASTOLIC (mmHg)	OXYGEN UPTAKE (ml/kg·min)
High	99	40	96	60	54.4
High	95	46	102	68	49.5
High	90	50	108	70	46.5
Above average	85	52	110	70	45.0
Above average	80	55	110	74	43.7
Above average	75	56	114	76	42.5
Above average	70	58	116	78	41.3
Average	65	59	118	80	41.0
Average	60	60	120	80	39.0
Average	55	62	120	80	39.0
Average	50	63	120	80	37.0
Average	45	64	122	80	37.0
Average	40	65	124	81	35.7
Average	35	67	126	84	35.7
Below average	30	68	130	85	34.6
Below average	25	70	130	88	33.5
Below average	20	72	132	90	32.9
Below average	15	74	138	90	31.5
Low	10	77	140	92	30.2
Low	5	82	146	100	27.1
Low	1	95	168	110	22.7
Population size		1538	1615	1615	1632
Average		63	123	81	37.5
Standard deviation		11.0	13.6	9.6	

[a]Data comes from the Cooper Clinic Coronary Risk Factor Profile Charts which are from data collected on patients being evaluated at the Cooper Clinic and standards being established at the Institute for Aerobics Research, Dallas, Texas. Published with permission.

TABLE A.5. (Continued) Physical fitness and health standards for men 30 to 39 years of age

MAXIMUM HEART RATE (beats/min)	CHOLES-TEROL (mg%)	TRIGLY-CERIDES (mg%)	GLUCOSE (mg%)	FAT (%)
210	135	35	75	7.1
204	158	50	85	11.1
200	169	60	89	13.4
200	175	67	91	14.8
198	182	75	94	16.2
196	188	80	95	17.2
194	193	87	96	18.2
192	197	93	99	19.2
191	203	100	100	20.1
190	208	105	100	21.1
189	215	113	102	22.0
188	220	120	104	22.8
186	224	129	105	23.6
184	230	140	105	24.4
183	235	150	107	25.5
181	240	169	110	26.4
180	250	187	110	28.0
177	256	207	114	29.8
174	271	241	115	32.2
168	289	324	120	36.0
150	340	756	133	45.9
1632	1387	1377	1376	1223
188	217	143	103	22.4
11.7	41.2	114.0	18.2	7.9

TABLE A.6. Physical fitness and health standards for men 40 to 49 years of age[a]

PERCENTILE RANKINGS		RESTING (SITTING)			MAXIMUM
		HEART RATE (beats/min)	BLOOD PRESSURE SYSTOLIC (mmHg)	DIASTOLIC (mmHg)	OXYGEN UPTAKE (ml/kg·min)
High	99	42	96	60	52.5
	95	47	104	70	48.0
	90	50	110	70	45.0
Above average	85	52	110	74	43.7
	80	54	111	76	42.5
	75	56	115	78	41.0
	70	58	118	80	40.0
Average	65	58	120	80	39.0
	60	60	120	80	37.0
	55	61	120	80	36.3
	50	62	121	80	35.7
	45	64	124	82	35.3
	40	65	126	84	34.3
	35	67	130	85	33.6
Below average	30	69	130	88	32.9
	25	71	131	90	31.5
	20	72	138	90	31.1
	15	75	140	92	30.2
Low	10	78	142	98	27.6
	5	84	150	100	24.1
	1	99	166	110	19.6
Population size		1826	1880	1880	1898
Average		64	124	83	36.0
Standard deviation		11.5	14.5	10.0	

[a]Data comes from the Cooper Clinic Coronary Risk Factor Profile Charts which are from data collected on patients being evaluated at the Cooper Clinic and standards being established at the Institute for Aerobics Research, Dallas, Texas. Published with permission.

TABLE A.6. (Continued) Physical fitness and health standards for men 40 to 49 years of age

MAXIMUM HEART RATE (beats/min)	CHOLES- TEROL (mg%)	TRIGLY- CERIDES (mg%)	GLUCOSE (mg%)	FAT (%)
205	145	37	80	9.2
200	165	53	87	13.0
196	175	63	90	14.9
193	186	72	93	16.6
191	193	78	95	17.7
190	199	85	97	18.8
188	204	91	99	19.7
186	209	98	100	20.7
185	214	105	101	21.5
183	220	112	103	22.2
182	225	121	105	23.0
180	230	130	105	23.8
180	235	139	107	24.6
178	240	150	109	25.4
176	245	162	110	26.3
174	250	180	111	27.4
171	257	200	114	28.5
168	265	227	115	30.0
164	275	269	120	32.2
158	295	363	125	36.1
139	338	590	160	44.4
1898	1681	1665	1662	1537
181	226	151	106	23.4
13.3	39.7	110.5	21.0	7.1

TABLE A.7. Physical fitness and health standards for men 50 to 59 years of age[a]

PERCENTILE RANKINGS		RESTING (SITTING)			MAXIMUM
		HEART RATE (beats/min)	BLOOD PRESSURE SYSTOLIC (mmHg)	DIASTOLIC (mmHg)	OXYGEN UPTAKE (ml/kg·min)
High	99	42	98	60	51.6
	95	47	108	70	45.4
	90	50	110	72	43.7
Above average	85	52	114	75	41.0
	80	55	116	78	39.0
	75	56	119	80	37.0
	70	58	120	80	36.0
Average	65	60	120	80	35.7
	60	60	122	80	34.6
	55	62	125	80	33.5
	50	63	128	82	32.9
	45	64	130	84	32.2
	40	65	130	86	31.5
	35	66	132	88	30.8
Below average	30	68	138	90	30.2
	25	70	140	90	29.2
	20	72	140	90	29.0
	15	75	144	95	26.2
Low	10	77	150	100	24.5
	5	82	160	102	21.0
	1	95	180	114	16.5
Population size		1046	1073	1073	1087
Average		63	129	84	33.6
Standard		11.0	17.2	10.4	

[a]Data comes from the Cooper Clinic Coronary Risk Factor Profile Charts which are from data collected on patients being evaluated at the Cooper Clinic and standards being established at the Institute for Aerobics Research, Dallas, Texas. Published with permission.

TABLE A.7. (Continued) Physical fitness and health standards for men 50 to 59 years of age

MAXIMUM HEART RATE (beats/min)	CHOLES-TEROL (mg%)	TRIGLY-CERIDES (mg%)	GLUCOSE (mg%)	FAT (%)
200	149	44	80	9.0
192	173	55	88	13.1
188	185	67	92	15.8
186	193	75	95	17.4
183	201	83	96	18.4
180	205	89	99	19.6
180	211	95	100	20.4
178	215	100	101	21.4
176	220	107	103	22.1
175	225	116	105	22.9
173	230	124	105	23.8
172	235	133	108	24.6
170	240	142	110	25.4
168	245	153	110	26.1
166	250	165	113	27.0
163	255	185	115	28.0
160	264	200	116	29.1
157	274	230	120	30.9
150	285	270	124	32.8
140	300	370	135	35.9
118	344	690	180	44.8
1087	942	936	935	847
171	233	157	108	24.1
15.9	40.5	120.9	21.2	7.0

TABLE A.8. Physical fitness and health standards for men 60+ years of age[a]

PERCENTILE RANKINGS		RESTING (SITTING)			MAXIMUM
		HEART RATE (beats/min)	BLOOD PRESSURE		OXYGEN UPTAKE (ml/kg·min)
			SYSTOLIC (mmHg)	DIASTOLIC (mmHg)	
High	99	38	98	60	49.5
	95	48	108	68	44.5
	90	52	112	70	41.0
Above average	85	54	118	72	36.6
	80	55	120	76	35.7
	75	56	120	78	35.0
	70	58	124	80	33.6
Average	65	58	128	80	32.2
	60	60	130	80	31.0
	55	60	130	80	30.2
	50	62	131	81	29.0
	45	64	135	84	29.0
	40	65	140	84	26.2
	35	67	140	86	25.9
Below average	30	68	140	88	24.5
	25	70	145	90	22.7
	20	72	150	90	21.8
	15	75	152	94	20.1
Low	10	77	160	98	17.5
	5	81	168	100	15.7
	1	94	184	118	14.0
Population size		267	275	275	279
Average		63	135	83	30.0
Standard deviation		10.4	18.3	11.0	

[a]Data comes from the Cooper Clinic Coronary Risk Factor Profile Charts which are from data collected on patients being evaluated at the Cooper Clinic and standards being established at the Institute for Aerobics Research, Dallas, Texas. Published with permission.

TABLE A.8. (Continued) Physical fitness and health standards for men 60+ years of age

MAXIMUM HEART RATE (beats/min)	CHOLES-TEROL (mg%)	TRIGLY-CERIDES (mg%)	GLUCOSE (mg%)	FAT (%)
195	152	43	83	10.5
186	173	55	89	12.3
184	180	66	92	14.1
180	190	73	94	16.2
175	196	76	96	17.2
172	201	82	100	18.0
170	205	89	102	18.9
170	210	95	104	19.9
165	214	100	105	20.8
163	217	106	106	21.5
162	225	115	108	22.3
160	228	122	110	23.3
159	234	129	110	24.4
156	240	142	112	25.4
152	250	150	115	26.9
148	256	160	118	28.0
145	264	170	120	28.9
140	268	195	124	30.1
131	280	233	129	32.5
121	291	291	140	35.6
104	345	552	170	42.4
249	243	241	241	211
159	228	139	110	23.1
19.5	39.1	99.4	23.4	7.2

TABLE A.9. Physical fitness and health standards for females 20 to 29 years of age[a]

PERCENTILE RANKINGS		RESTING (SITTING)			MAXIMUM
		HEART RATE (beats/min)	BLOOD PRESSURE SYSTOLIC (mmHg)	DIASTOLIC (mmHg)	OXYGEN UPTAKE (ml/kg·min)
High	99	48	90	56	45.0
	95	52	97	60	41.0
	90	55	100	63	38.0
Above average	85	58	100	65	37.0
	80	59	101	68	35.7
	75	60	105	70	34.3
	70	60	106	70	33.6
Average	65	62	110	70	32.9
	60	63	110	72	31.5
	55	64	110	74	30.9
	50	65	112	75	30.2
	45	68	115	75	30.0
	40	70	118	78	29.6
	35	70	118	78	29.2
Below average	30	72	120	80	29.0
	25	74	120	80	27.6
	20	75	120	80	25.3
	15	80	122	80	24.0
Low	10	84	130	82	21.8
	5	86	140	88	20.4
	1	100	141	90	19.2
Population size		115	118	118	119
Average		67	114	74	31.1
Standard deviation		11.2	12.0	7.8	

[a]Data comes from the Cooper Clinic Coronary Risk Factor Profile Charts which are from data collected on patients being evaluated at the Cooper Clinic and standards being established at the Institute for Aerobics Research, Dallas, Texas. Published with permission.

TABLE A.9. (Continued) Physical fitness and health standards for females 20 to 20 years of age

MAXIMUM HEART RATE (beats/min)	CHOLES-TEROL (mg%)	TRIGLY-CERIDES (mg%)	GLUCOSE (mg%)	FAT (%)
213	135	30	56	4.8
208	144	43	75	6.6
203	150	45	81	11.6
199	160	47	85	14.5
198	165	50	86	15.1
196	170	52	87	16.1
194	170	58	90	18.3
192	174	60	92	20.2
190	182	65	94	23.2
190	185	72	94	24.1
188	190	76	95	24.9
187	195	81	97	25.6
186	196	88	99	26.2
184	200	107	99	27.3
182	210	109	100	28.2
181	215	120	100	30.3
180	219	126	101	33.3
174	224	138	103	36.4
172	251	158	105	38.5
168	265	235	115	45.5
160	380	635	200	62.9
119	68	68	67	61
188	195	102	96	25.0
11.8	41.8	89.7	20.9	11.5

TABLE A.10. Physical fitness and health standards for females 30 to 39 years of age[a]

| PERCENTILE RANKINGS | | RESTING (SITTING) | | | MAXIMUM |
		HEART RATE (beats/min)	BLOOD PRESSURE SYSTOLIC (mmHg)	DIASTOLIC (mmHg)	OXYGEN UPTAKE (ml/kg·min)
High	99	48	90	60	43.7
	95	52	98	60	40.0
	90	55	100	65	37.0
Above average	85	57	100	70	35.7
	80	58	104	70	35.0
	75	60	106	70	33.6
	70	62	110	70	32.9
Average	65	62	110	71	31.5
	60	65	110	74	31.5
	55	66	110	75	30.2
	50	68	114	76	30.2
	45	68	116	80	29.3
	40	70	118	80	29.0
	35	72	120	80	27.6
Below average	30	74	120	80	26.2
	25	75	120	80	25.7
	20	76	122	82	24.5
	15	80	125	85	23.1
Low	10	82	130	90	21.7
	5	85	140	90	21.0
	1	108	160	110	17.0
Population size		280	301	301	309
Average		68	115	77	30.3
Standard deviation		11.5	13.3	9.9	

[a]Data comes from the Cooper Clinic Coronary Risk Factor Profile Charts which are from data collected on patients being evaluated at the Cooper Clinic and standards being established at the Institute for Aerobics Research, Dallas, Texas. Published with permission.

TABLE A.10. (Continued) Physical fitness and health standards for females 30 to 39 years of age

MAXIMUM				
HEART RATE (beats/min)	**CHOLES-TEROL** (mg%)	**TRIGLY-CERIDES** (mg%)	**GLUCOSE** (mg%)	**FAT** (%)
210	124	25	60	5.1
200	141	37	79	10.1
196	158	44	83	13.1
194	165	48	85	14.8
192	168	51	88	16.7
190	172	55	90	18.3
189	176	59	91	19.3
187	184	62	92	20.5
185	188	68	95	21.5
185	191	73	95	22.5
184	195	77	95	23.6
183	200	80	97	24.6
182	204	85	99	25.5
180	206	88	100	26.3
180	211	93	100	27.6
178	218	100	101	29.0
176	224	108	103	31.3
174	231	120	105	34.6
170	240	132	107	38.1
164	255	157	111	42.9
148	300	428	116	68.6
309	220	220	220	192
183	197	89	95	24.8
14.8	36.0	68.0	14.8	11.0

TABLE A.11. Physical fitness and health standards for females 40 to 49 years of age[a]

PERCENTILE RANKINGS		RESTING (SITTING)			MAXIMUM
		HEART RATE (beats/min)	BLOOD PRESSURE		OXYGEN UPTAKE (ml/kg·min)
			SYSTOLIC (mmHg)	DIASTOLIC (mmHg)	
High	99	43	90	58	43.7
	95	52	100	60	37.0
	90	55	100	65	35.0
Above average	85	58	102	70	32.9
	80	60	105	70	31.5
	75	60	110	70	30.9
	70	62	110	70	30.2
Average	65	63	110	74	30.2
	60	64	112	75	29.0
	55	65	114	78	29.0
	50	66	118	80	26.7
	45	68	120	80	26.2
	40	70	120	80	25.3
	35	72	120	80	24.5
Below average	30	72	120	80	24.5
	25	74	124	80	22.9
	20	76	130	82	22.7
	15	80	132	86	21.0
Low	10	80	138	90	21.0
	5	87	150	94	19.2
	1	100	164	110	15.7
Population size		260	282	282	286
Average		68	118	78	28.0
Standard dveiation		10.7	15.7	10.2	

[a]Data comes from the Cooper Clinic Coronary Risk Factor Profile Charts which are from data collected on patients being evaluated at the Cooper Clinic and standards being established at the Institute for Aerobics Research, Dallas, Texas. Published with permission.

TABLE A.11. (Continued) Physical fitness and health standards for females 40 to 49 years of age

MAXIMUM HEART RATE (beats/min)	CHOLES-TEROL (mg%)	TRIGLY-CERIDES (mg%)	GLUCOSE (mg%)	FAT (%)
208	130	35	75	7.3
196	158	45	82	12.0
192	171	49	86	15.8
189	178	56	88	17.9
186	184	58	90	19.6
185	190	63	91	21.0
183	195	67	92	21.9
180	198	73	94	22.7
180	201	77	95	23.9
178	205	82	95	24.9
177	210	86	96	25.9
175	213	91	98	26.7
173	217	98	100	27.6
172	223	105	100	28.2
170	228	110	100	29.1
169	235	118	104	30.2
166	241	130	105	31.4
162	252	148	107	33.7
158	264	162	111	37.4
148	283	223	117	43.1
133	319	450	153	49.7
286	218	216	215	183
175	214	106	98	26.1
14.8	39.4	89.9	16.6	8.6

TABLE A.12. Physical fitness and health standards for females 50 to 59 years of age[a]

PERCENTILE RANKINGS		RESTING (SITTING)			MAXIMUM
		HEART RATE (beats/min)	BLOOD PRESSURE SYSTOLIC (mmHg)	DIASTOLIC (mmHg)	OXYGEN UPTAKE (ml/kg·min)
High	99	45	90	58	52.5
	95	52	100	64	35.7
	90	55	108	69	32.9
Above average	85	58	110	70	31.5
	80	60	110	70	30.2
	75	60	115	74	30.2
	70	61	118	75	29.0
Average	65	62	120	76	27.6
	60	64	120	79	26.2
	55	65	120	80	25.3
	50	67	122	80	24.5
	45	68	128	80	24.5
	40	69	130	82	23.6
	35	70	130	84	22.7
Below average	30	72	134	85	22.7
	25	74	140	88	21.9
	20	75	140	90	21.0
	15	78	142	90	20.4
Low	10	83	148	92	19.2
	5	89	160	100	17.6
	1	105	172	110	14.4
Population size		162	167	167	169
Average		68	126	80	25.7
Standard deviation		11.7	16.8	10.6	

[a]Data comes from the Cooper Clinic Coronary Risk Factor Profile Charts which are from data collected on patients being evaluated at the Cooper Clinic and standards being established at the Institute for Aerobics Research, Dallas, Texas. Published with permission.

TABLE A.12. (Continued) Physical fitness and health standards for females 50 to 59 years of age

MAXIMUM HEART RATE (beats/min)	CHOLES-TEROL (mg%)	TRIGLY-CERIDES (mg%)	GLUCOSE (mg%)	FAT (%)
202	158	39	78	10.8
190	170	50	85	15.9
185	180	60	89	18.2
182	192	68	91	21.0
180	198	70	93	22.7
179	202	77	95	23.9
176	205	82	95	25.1
174	214	91	97	26.1
173	218	98	99	27.0
172	221	105	100	27.7
170	225	110	100	28.4
168	230	115	102	29.6
167	234	118	105	30.4
164	236	125	105	31.4
162	241	130	108	32.5
160	249	145	110	33.4
160	260	165	110	34.7
156	267	175	111	37.1
152	275	218	115	39.7
144	295	242	120	44.4
128	320	395	135	61.2
169	137	136	137	127
169	228	123	102	29.3
14.5	27.3	67.1	15.1	9.5

TABLE A.13. Physical fitness and health standards for females 60+ years of age[a]

PERCENTILE RANKINGS		RESTING (SITTING)			MAXIMUM
		HEART RATE (beats/min)	BLOOD PRESSURE SYSTOLIC (mmHg)	DIASTOLIC (mmHg)	OXYGEN UPTAKE (ml/kg·min)
High	99	46	110	66	37.0
	95	50	118	70	31.5
	90	52	120	70	30.2
Above average	85	56	120	71	30.2
	80	57	120	75	26.9
	75	59	122	75	25.3
	70	60	125	76	25.3
Average	65	60	125	78	24.5
	60	62	128	80	24.5
	55	64	130	80	23.9
	50	64	130	80	21.8
	45	64	132	80	21.3
	40	66	136	80	21.0
	35	70	139	81	20.1
Below average	30	72	140	84	20.1
	25	72	140	86	19.2
	20	74	142	88	18.3
	15	75	150	90	17.5
Low	10	79	160	98	16.1
	5	80	165	100	15.7
	1	85	188	100	12.3
Population size		43	46	46	46
Average		65	135	81	22.9
Standard deviation		9.6	16.2	8.8	

[a]Data comes from the Cooper Clinic Coronary Risk Factor Profile Charts which are from data collected on patients being evaluated at the Cooper Clinic and standards being established at the Institute for Aerobics Research, Dallas, Texas. Published with permission.

TABLE A.13. (Continued) Physical fitness and health standards for females 60+ years of age

MAXIMUM				
HEART RATE (beats/min)	**CHOLES-TEROL** (mg%)	**TRIGLY-CERIDES** (mg%)	**GLUCOSE** (mg%)	**FAT** (%)
178	127	42	75	6.8
178	180	46	80	13.1
176	185	62	88	17.7
170	188	72	90	19.3
165	210	80	91	22.2
162	220	87	94	24.0
160	223	90	97	25.1
158	235	93	98	26.6
155	235	97	100	27.1
155	238	105	100	27.9
153	240	110	102	29.8
151	245	124	104	30.4
150	245	129	105	30.8
150	246	134	107	31.2
145	262	140	110	31.7
142	265	164	110	32.5
140	269	183	110	34.7
128	275	210	110	35.2
126	276	228	115	36.3
120	310	277	120	39.9
106	335	400	130	51.2
46	40	39	39	32
151	237	131	102	28.3
17.5	40.9	71.5	14.9	8.5

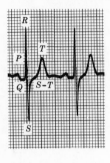

(a)

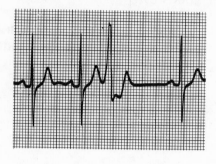

(b)

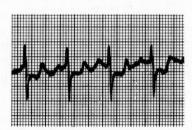

(c)

FIGURE A.1. *(a)* The deflections in a normal ECG are the P wave (atrial depolarization), QRS complex (ventricular depolarization), and T wave (ventricular repolarization). The S-T segment is the interval between the end of the QRS complex and the beginning of the T wave. *(b)* An ECG with a premature ventricular beat. *(c)* An ECG with 2 millimeters S-T segment depression.

If proper guidelines for exercise tolerance testing are followed, in which symptoms, signs, ECG, and blood pressure monitoring are included, specific changes will guide the tester as to when the safety of the test subject may be in question. The problem with using submaximal exercise tests and, in particular, ones that bring the heart rate up to a range of only 150 beats per minute is that they are subject to gross errors in predicting cardiorespiratory fitness and would not generally bring the participant's heart rate up to the level at which he or she is training. Maximum heart rate is quite variable from one individual to another and can range from 140 to over 200 beats per minute for a healthy 50-year-old. Therefore, if a tester were to use an arbitrary cutoff point of 85 percent of predicted maximum heart rate then, in fact, the participant could be stressed to 100 percent of capacity or only 60 percent. Our experience has shown that most sedentary middle-aged men beginning a jogging program train at heart rates ranging from 70 to 90 percent of maximum heart rate range (approximately 150 to 185 beats per minute.

Although many laboratories use 85 percent of predicted maximum heart rate as an automatic cutoff point for termination of a test, the more recent trend in exercise tolerance testing has been to continue the test until a person has symptoms or fatigue. This end point is termed functional maximum capacity. Also, evidence exists suggesting that many persons do not show ECG abnormalities until their heart rate is above 85 percent of maximum; hence the submaximal screening test is considered less sensitive as a diagnostic tool. A recent study conducted at the Aerobics Institute, Dallas, Texas, showed that of the 7059 males who were administered a maximal exercise test, approximately 15 percent were considered abnormal or questionable. Among the 552 abnormal tests, 34 percent *did not* become abnormal until after the heart rate exceeded 85 percent of predicted maximum heart rate.

During an exercise test the safety of the participant is of the utmost importance and yet, taking one to functional maximum has not been shown to be any more dangerous than the 85 percent heart rate cutoff point. The secret to the safety of the test is to have good monitoring of the participant and to have highly trained personnel administering the test. Even in hospital settings, where many patients are referred with suspicions of coronary heart disease, the mortality rate has been shown to be 1 per 10,000 exercise tests. With the availability of resuscitation equipment (including defibrillator) and trained personnel, most of these individuals should be resuscitated without further complications. The aforementioned results are based mainly on a middle-aged population in which coronary heart disease was suspected. The rate for young persons would be more favorable.

The *end point* for termination of a maximum stress test is dependent upon when a participant reaches volitional exhaustion or when any of the following "indications for stopping" occur.

1. Failure of monitoring system.

2. Progressive angina (chest discomfort or pain).

3. Two-millimeter horizontal or downsloping ST depression on ECG. (As long as a patient is not having symptoms, some laboratories will not use this as a terminating point).

4. Sustained supraventricular tachycardia.

5. Ventricular tachycardia.

6. Exercise induced left or right bundle branch block.

7. Any significant drop (10 millimeters of mercury) in systolic blood pressure.

8. Light headedness, confusion, ataxia, pallor, cyanosis, nausea, or any sign of peripheral circulatory insufficiency.

9. Inappropriate bradycardia (slow heart rate).

10. Excessive blood pressure: systolic greater than 260 millimeters of mercury, diastolic greater than 120 millimeters of mercury.

11. Presence of dangerous dysrhythmias (irregular heart beats) such as frequent premature ventricular contractions (PVC's) and multifocal PVC's (premature beats that are triggered from more than one area of the heart).

Heart rate, blood pressure, and ECG monitoring should continue at a regular basis during and in recovery from an exercise test. At minimum, these variables should be recorded every three minutes during exercise, at maximum or immediately after cessation of exercise, and at one, three, and five minutes during recovery. If abnormalities in the ECG occur, more frequent tracings are required, or in serious cases, they should be monitored continuously. See Table A.14 for an example of a stress test data recording form.

How many different ECG leads should be monitored during a stress test? This is an interesting question and is beyond the scope of this book. In general though, a single bipolar lead system (two electrodes) is not adequate for diagnostic purposes. A multilead system of up to 15 leads gives the most accurate diagnosis. For example, the above mentioned study conducted at the Aerobics Institute also showed the importance of doing *multilead* monitoring during an exercise test. In this study, 22 percent of the men who showed significant ST segment depression did not have an abnormal test in lead V_5 (the most common chest lead used in exercise testing). For more details on this subject see the text by Ellestad.

Exercise testing can be administered on a motorized treadmill (high expense), bicycle ergometer (medium expense), or stepping bench (low cost). For low-risk younger persons who have had some training experience, a 12-minute or 1.5-mile run can be used to estimate maximum oxygen uptake. Although each mode of testing has its advantages and disadvantages, for persons not used to bicycle riding, the treadmill type test is most preferred. The 12-minute or 1.5-mile run field test should never be used as a diagnostic test for the determination of the presence or absence of disease. Usually, all diagnostic tests should meet the same general criteria for work load and progression when used to determine functional capacity and status of health. These criteria are listed under treadmill protocols.

MAXIMAL EXERCISE TOLERANCE TEST PROTOCOLS

Treadmill protocols.   There are many maximal exercise tolerance test protocols in use today, and no one test is thought to be superior. Certain guidelines to consider when selecting a test protocol would include the following:

1. The test should be graded with the initial work load not exceeding 2 to 3½ METS.* An exception to this would be if the test were not being used for diagnostic purposes and when the participants are of low risk.

2. The progressive increases in work load should not exceed 1 MET

---

* MET refers to metabolic equivalent above the resting metabolic level. One MET (resting value) is equal to approximately 3.5 milliliters per kilogram of body weight per minute of oxygen consumed.

TABLE A.14. Stress Test Summary*

STRESS TEST SUMMARY

INSTITUTE FOR AEROBICS RESEARCH

PATIENT NO.

B.T.X - ___ - ___

VISIT ___   FORM ___ Q

Name: _____
Last Name First   Kg [1]
                      lb. [2]

Date: ___ / ___ / ___
MONTH   DAY   YR.

Age: ___ Body Wt: ___   Cm [1]
                          In [2]   Ht: ___   Sex: ☐   Group: ___

Bar. Pr. ___ mm   Time ___   Leads: 5 [1]
                             AM [1]   7 [2]
Humidity ___ %   PM [2]   10 [3]

Resting:

	H.R.	Blood Pressure
Supine	___	___ / ___
Sitting	___	___ / ___
Standing	___	___ / ___

Test Type:
Balke [1]
Bruce [2]
Elstad [3]
Astrand [4]
Ergometer [5]
Other [6]

Comments: _____
_____
_____
_____
_____

Warm Up:

Treadmill [1]   Ergometer [2]

A. Kpm-mph ___
   % Grade ___
   Minutes ___
B. Kpm-mph ___
   % Grade ___
   Minutes ___

End of Test:

Total time = ___ : ___
Max H.R. = ___
Max B.P. = ___ / ___

Reasons For Stopping:

Nausea [3]	Leg Weakness [6]	Hypotension [9]
Anxiety [1]	Dizziness [4]	Claudication [7]	ECG Changes [A]
Dyspnea [2]	Chest Pain [5]	Gen. Fatigue [8]	Hypertension [B]

Other [C] _____
_____

Codes: W = Warm Up, E = Exercise, R = Recovery

Code	Time	H.R.	Blood Pressure	Load or Speed Kpm - mph	Grade	Temp.	Vent. (ATPS)	% O₂	% CO₂
☐	_:_	__	_/_	__	__	_._	_._	_._	_._
☐	_:_	__	_/_	__	__	_._	_._	_._	_._
☐	_:_	__	_/_	__	__	_._	_._	_._	_._
☐	_:_	__	_/_	__	__	_._	_._	_._	_._
☐	_:_	__	_/_	__	__	_._	_._	_._	_._
☐	_:_	__	_/_	__	__	_._	_._	_._	_._
☐	_:_	__	_/_	__	__	_._	_._	_._	_._
☐	_:_	__	_/_	__	__	_._	_._	_._	_._
☐	_:_	__	_/_	__	__	_._	_._	_._	_._
☐	_:_	__	_/_	__	__	_._	_._	_._	_._
☐	_:_	__	_/_	__	__	_._	_._	_._	_._
☐	_:_	__	_/_	__	__	_._	_._	_._	_._
☐	_:_	__	_/_	__	__	_._	_._	_._	_._
☐	_:_	__	_/_	__	__	_._	_._	_._	_._
☐	_:_	__	_/_	__	__	_._	_._	_._	_._

*Published with permission of the Institute for Aerobics Research, Dallas, Texas.

per increase in increment for high-risk patients and 2 to 3 METS for low-risk patients.

3. For continuous tests each work load should be performed for at least one minute before increasing to the next work load.

4. The initial phase of recovery should be with the participant either in the supine position or continuing to exercise at a very low level of work. On a treadmill, the latter would mean walking at 2 miles per hour, 0 percent grade; on a bicycle ergometer, it would mean pedalling 50 to 60 revolutions per minute at little or no resistance; and, after a bench step test, moving the legs back and forth while in place. If a person stops and immediately sits down after exercise, the blood tends to pool in the lower extremities and the person could become faint (vasomotor hypotension). This condition could be particularly hazardous with diseased individuals.

Table A.14 is an example of an exercise tolerance test data collection form. Figure A.2 shows an example of three popularly used maximal treadmill exercise test protocols. Figure A.3 best describes the differences in the three protocols. The time duration and rate of increase in oxygen cost (METS) differs significantly between tests, while the end result (maximum oxygen uptake) is approximately the same.

In reviewing the guidelines for a stress test mentioned above, the Bruce and Balke protocols meet the criteria for a diagnostic test, while the modified Åstrand test starts out at too high an energy cost level. The latter test is strictly a running protocol and is best used to evaluate experienced runners and athletes to determine their maximum oxygen uptake. The biggest criticism of the Balke test is the time involved in completing the test, while the Bruce protocol is criticized for its abrupt changes in work loads. Whatever the case, both the Bruce and Balke tests have been used successfully with groups of varying ability, body type, age, and health status.

In using the Balke test, if the treadmill being used is limited to a maximum elevation of 25 percent, the speed will be increased by 0.2 mile per hour increments every minute after the 25th minute.

The modified Åstrand test is usually preceeded by a five-minute warm-up walk or jog. For beginners, a 3.5 mile per hour walk at 2.5-percent grade has worked well. The speed of the test is then adjusted to exhaust the participant within a 7- to 10-minute period. This time period is considered adequate for maximal physiological adjustments to occur. Table 3.3 shows the recommended speed of running to be used

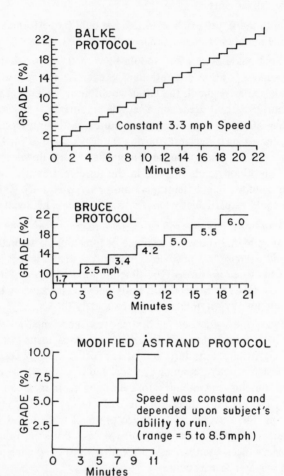

FIGURE A.2. Maximal exercise tolerance test protocols for Balke, Bruce, and Åstrand.

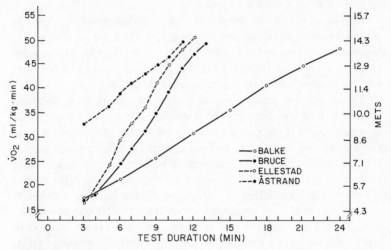

FIGURE A.3. Rate of increase in oxygen untake in four stress test protocols on 51 men, aged 35 to 55 years. From Pollock *et al.* "A comparative analysis of four protocols for maximal treadmill stress testing." *Am. Heart J.* 92:39-46 (1976).

with persons of varying abilities.Therefore, the speed of the test can be estimated by knowing a person's Balke or Bruce treadmill time or one-and-one-half mile run time.

Examples of three other popularly used treadmill stress protocols are shown in Tables A.15 to A.17. These protocols (Kattus, Naughton, and Wilson) begin at a lower MET level than the Bruce or Balke test and are often used with cardiac patients.

Bicycle and Step Test Protocols. Although the mode of testing is different with a bicycle or step test protocol, the rules are the same as compared to the treadmill protocols. The most popular maximal bicycle test has been adapted from Åstrand. The test is a continuous, multistage protocol to maximal volitional exhaustion.

The bicycle test requires a good quality bicycle ergometer in which the work load can be precisely measured. Work load on a bicycle ergometer is usually expressed in kilopond meters of work per minute (kpm/min). For women, the test would begin at 300 kpm/min and for men at approximately 600 kpm/min. After each two to three minute increment, the work load is increased 150 kilopond meters per minute for women and 300 kilopond meters per minute for men. If the gradation of the work load on the ergometer is not in 150 kilopond meter per minute increments, a 100 kilopond meter per minute increase in work load every two minutes will be satisfactory for women; that is, most bicycle ergometers are graded in increments of 100 or 150 kilopond meters per minute.

Many bicycles do not internally adjust the work load to compensate for change in pedalling rate; therefore, in this case, one would have to pedal at a constant rate, that is, revolution per minute (rpm). For the test described above, a pedal rate of 50 revolutions per minute is recommended. In this case, a metronome will assist the participant in keeping the proper pedal speed. Also, frequent calibration of all mechanical type bicycles is important. The friction type is the easiest to calibrate. With this type of bicycle, the friction belt expands as heat is generated by the fly wheel, and thus periodic tightening of the belt corrects for change in work load.

Another important point to remember when using a bicycle ergometer is to make sure the height of the seat is properly adjusted. The seat should be adjusted so that there is a slight bend in the knee joint with the ball of the foot on the pedal when the pedal is in its lowest position.

TABLE A.15. Kattus treadmill test[a]

I. PRELIMINARY DATA

SUBJECT _____

Resting Heart Rate _____ Resting Blood Pressure _____

Age _____ Test Administrator(s) _____

II. GRADED EXERCISE TEST

STAGE	DURATION (min)	TIME (min)	SPEED (mph and m/min)	GRADE (%)	METS	HEART RATE	BLOOD PRESSURE
1	3	1-3	1.5 40.2	10	4.22		
2	3	4-6	2.0 53.6	10	5.29		
3	3	7-9	2.5 67.0	10	6.36		
4	3	10-12	3.0 80.5	10	7.43		
5	3	13-15	3.5 93.8	10	8.50		
6	3	16-19	4.0 107.3	10	9.58		
END OF SUBMAXIMAL EXERCISE							
7	3	20.23	4.0 107.3	14	11.79		
8	3	24-27	4.0 107.3	18	14		
9	3	28-31	4.0 107.3	22	16.2		
RECOVERY		2 minutes	Sitting				
		4 minutes	Sitting				
		6 minutes	Sitting				
		8 minutes	Sitting				

COMMENTS:

[a]Kattus, A.A. "Physical Training and Beta-adrenergic Blocking Drugs in Modifying Coronary Insufficiency." Marchetti, G. and B. Toccardi (editors), *Coronary Circulation and Energetics of the Myocardium*, Karger, New York, 1967.

TABLE A.16. Naughton treadmill test[a]

I. PRELIMINARY DATA

SUBJECT _____

Resting Heart Rate _____   Resting Blood Pressure _____

Age _____   Test Administrator(s) _____

II. GRADED EXERCISE TEST

STAGE	DURATION (min)	TIME (min)	SPEED (mph and m/min)		GRADE (%)	METS	HEART RATE	BLOOD PRESSURE
1	2	1-2	1	26.8	0	1.77		
2	2	3-4	2.0	53.6	0	2.53		
3	2	5-6	2.0	53.6	3.5	3.5		
4	2	7-8	2.0	53.6	7.0	4.46		
5	2	9-10	2.0	53.6	10.5	5.43		
6	2	11-12	2.0	53.6	14	6.39		
7	2	13-14	2.0	53.6	17.5	7.36		
RECOVERY		2 minutes	Sitting					
		4 minutes	Sitting					
		6 minutes	Sitting					
		8 minutes	Sitting					

COMMENTS:

[a]Naughton, J., B. Balke, and F. Nagle. "Refinements in Methods of Evaluation and Physical Conditioning Before and After Myocardial Infarction." *Am. J. Card., 14*:837 (1964).

TABLE A.17. Wilson (functional) treadmill test (Beginning)[a]

I. PRELIMINARY DATA

SUBJECT _____

Resting Heart Rate _____ Resting Blood Pressure _____

Age _____ Test Administrator(s) _____

II. GRADED EXERCISE TEST

STAGE	DURATION (min)	TIME (min)	SPEED (mph and m/min)		GRADE (%)	METS	HEART RATE	BLOOD PRESSURE
1	3	1-3	1.5	40.2	0	2.15	_____	_____
2	3	4-6	2.0	53.6	0	2.53	_____	_____
3	3	7-9	2.5	67.0	0	2.91	_____	_____
4	3	10-12	3.0	80.5	0	3.30	_____	_____
5	3	13-15	3.0	80.5	5	5.36		
6	3	16-18	3.0	80.5	7.5	6.39		
7	3	19-21	3.0	80.5	10	7.43		
RECOVERY		2 minutes	Sitting				_____	_____
		4 minutes	Sitting				_____	_____
		6 minutes	Sitting				_____	_____
		8 minutes	Sitting				_____	_____

COMMENTS:

[a]Wilson, P.K., E.R. Winga, J.W. Edgett, and T.J. Gushiken, *Policies and Procedures of a Cardiac Rehabilitation Program—Immediate to Long Term Care.* Philadelphia: Lea & Febiger Co., 1978.

In comparison to a treadmill, there are some advantages in using the bicycle ergometer. It is much less expensive and is somewhat portable. It has obvious advantages if one is testing in more than one location. There is less upper body movement in bicycle testing, and thus blood pressure is easier to assess. This is particularly true at the higher work levels. And finally, in some cases, ECG recordings may show less skeletal muscle interference with bicycle ergometry.

The major disadvantage of bicycle testing is that most Americans are unaccustomed to bicycle riding; hence their maximal values (heart rate and maximum oxygen uptake) are often underestimated. The underestimation can range from 5 to 25 percent, depending upon the participant's conditioning and leg strength. Since an underestimation of functional capacity has obvious limitations in evaluation and exercise prescription, most testers prefer to use the treadmill.

A recommended *step test* would include a stepping bench that can be automatically adjusted in height from 2 to 50 centimeters (1 in. = 2.54 cm). The stepping rate for the test is 30 per minute and it begins at a height of 2 centimeters with an increase of 2 centimeters each minute thereafter. At the count of one-two, the participant steps up on the platform until completely erect with both feet on the platform. Counts three-four will bring the participant back down to the starting position. To help avoid muscle fatigue, the participant can change the lead leg at any time. To help keep the proper stepping rhythm, the use of a metronome is recommended. The test is terminated at volitional fatigue or when the participant cannot keep up the proper rhythm.

SUBMAXIMAL EXERCISE TOLERANCE TEST PROTOCOLS TO DETERMINE MAXIMUM FUNCTIONAL CAPACITY

The second category of exercise testing listed in Table 3.2, Plan B, is termed submaximal testing to estimate maximum functional capacity. Often the tests are similar to those described under maximal stress testing except that the test is terminated at some predetermined submaximal heart rate level. These protocols require the same careful preliminary precautions and ECG and blood pressure monitoring during exercise and recovery as described for the maximal test.

The submaximal testing protocols normally predict maximum functional capacity (maximum oxygen uptake) from heart rate response. Heart rate and oxygen uptake increase linearly in response to added

Table A.18. Maximum heart rate, percent maximum heart rate, and percent maximum heart rate range by age.

Condition	Age (yr)					
	20	30	40	50	60	70
Max HR[a]	201	193	186	179	172	165
85% Max HR	171	164	158	152	146	140
85% Max HR Range[b]	181	175	169	163	157	151
70% Max HR	141	135	130	125	120	115
70% Max HR Range[b]	162	156	151	146	142	137

[a]Maximum heart rate as determined by Cooper and others.
[b]Percent of maximum heart rate range as determined by Karvonen. Calculation assumes a resting heart rate of 70 beats per minute.

work and thus a general extrapolation can be made to predict maximum capacity. Although this method of predicting functional capacity is used by some testers, it has definite limitations. First, because of the variability of maximum heart rate, the estimation of maximum oxygen uptake from submaximal heart rate has been shown to have a standard error of approximately plus or minus 10 percent. Also, this type of test tends to overestimate for highly trained persons and underestimate for unfit persons. Therefore, this potential error must be considered in the interpretation of test results and the exercise prescription. Second, and most important, if a submaximal test is used for diagnostic purposes, the testee should only be given clearance up to that point. As mentioned previously, significant ECG and/or blood pressure abnormalities often occur at heart rates above 85 percent of predicted maximum. Since jogging, running, and other moderate to high intensity training programs may be performed at heart rates higher than this, the practice of evaluating individuals at submaximal levels is not sound. Thus, as mentioned earlier in this chapter, the evaluation of a participant to a symptom limited maximum is highly recommended.

Submaximal Treadmill Test. The use of either the Balke or Bruce tests (Figure A.2) is recommended as a submaximal treadmill stress test. The only difference between protocols described under maximal and submaximal tests would be the cutoff point. Unless symptoms occur, the termination of the test would be at 85 percent of predicted heart rate range.

If actual maximum heart rate is not known, use the value corresponding to age as shown in Table A.18. To determine 85 percent of maximum heart rate range the participant should also take into account the resting heart rate. The idea is to find 85 percent of the range between resting and maximum. To calculate, first subtract the resting heart rate from the maximum. Multiply this difference by 0.85. Then take this value and add to the resting heart rate. For example, if a person was 40 years of age and had a resting heart rate of 70 beats per minute, 70 would be subtracted from 186. The value 116 would then be multiplied by 0.85. The answer, 99, would then be added to 70. Thus, the value of 169 beats per minute would be used as the target heart rate.

Some testers calculate the target heart rate by taking 85 percent of the maximum heart rate. In the example above, 186 would be multiplied by 0.85. This would result in a target heart rate of 158 beats per minute, 11 beats per minute lower than the maximum heart rate range technique. The first method, which takes resting heart rate into consideration, is more accurate in its relationship to oxygen uptake. The latter technique tends to underestimate the actual oxygen uptake value, and therefore could lead to an inaccurate exercise prescription. If the prescription or target heart rate does not have to be based on oxygen cost (METS) then either technique can be used. For further determinations of percent of maximum heart rate (85 and 70 percent) and its comparison to percent of maximum heart rate from ages 20 to 70, see Table A.18.

Once the target heart rate is established, then the test will proceed as described above. Monitoring will be as described under maximal tests.

To predict maximum oxygen uptake from the submaximal test, follow these procedures:

1. Find the oxygen uptake (MET) equivalent to the time performed on the treadmill up to 85 percent of maximum heart rate range Table (3.3).

2. Multiply this value by 0.174.

3. Add this answer to the original value found in 1.

For example, if a person reached the target heart rate after eight minutes on a Bruce test (85% of maximum), the initial value for oxygen uptake would be 24.5 milliliters per kilogram of body weight per minute (7.0 METS). Multiply 24.5 (or 7.0) by 0.174. Take this answer (4.3 millileters per kilogram of body weight per minute, or 1.2 METS) and add to 24.5 (or 7.0). Thus, the estimated maximum oxygen uptake would be 28.8 millileters per kilogram of body weight per minute (or 8.2 METS).

Submaximal Bicycle Test. If a treadmill test is not desired, a continuous, multistage, submaximal bicycle test can be used to predict one's maximum oxygen uptake. Like the treadmill test, the bicycle test uses the heart rate response at different work loads to make this prediction. The assumption of this test is that heart rate and oxygen uptake are linear functions of work rate; thus, an adequate estimation can be made.

Once a participant has had a chance to become familiar with the bicycle and the proper seat height has been adjusted, then the test can start. As was described for the maximal bicycle protocol, set the metronome so that one can pedal at 50 revolutions per minute and let the testee warm-up by pedalling for one minute at zero work load. The test consists of a series of three minute work bouts that progress higher in load and at a level dependent on the participant's ability (heart rate response). The test is designed to begin at 300 kilopond meters per minute of work. Figure A.4 outlines the exact procedures of progression in the submaximal bicycle test. Each work load is timed for three minutes with the heart rate being counted during the last half of the second and third minutes. At the end of each heart rate count, the scores are recorded on a form such as the one shown in Table A.19. The heart rate in the second and third minutes should not differ by more than 5 beats per min. If they do, extend the test period for an additional minute or until a stable value is maintained.

To determine the next work load, check the heart rate value for the third minute of the initial work load. If the heart rate is less than 90 beats per minute, set the next work load at 900 kilopond meters per minute, if it is between 90 and 105 beats per minute, set the next work load at 750 kilopond meters per minute; and, if it is higher than 105 beats per minute, set the work load at 600 kilopond meters per minute. The same procedure is used for counting and recording heart rate as described for the initial work load. The guide for setting the final work

TABLE A.19. Worksheet for use in determining maximum oxygen uptake on submaximal test

NAME _____ AGE _____ WEIGHT _____ LB _____ KG

DATE

	Second Load HR[a]	Third Load HR	Maximum Work Load	Maximum Oxygen Uptake (L/min)	Maximum Oxygen Uptake (ml/kg)
Test 1	____ / ____	_____	_____	_____	_____
Test 2	____ / ____	_____	_____	_____	_____
Test 3	____ / ____	_____	_____	_____	_____

Directions	HR										HR
1. Plot the heart rate of the second and third loads versus the work (kpm/min)	200										200
	190										190
2. Determine maximum heart rate line from information on Table A.18.	180										180
	170										170

3. Draw a line through both points and extend to the maximum heart rate line for age.

4. Drop a line from this point to the baseline and read the maximum oxygen uptake.

| | 160 | 150 | 140 | 130 | 120 | 110 | 100 | 90 |

WORKLOAD (kpm/min)	300	450	600	750	900	1050	1200	1350	1500	1650	1800	1950	2100
MAXIMUM OXYGEN UPTAKE (L/m)	0.9	1.2	1.5	1.8	2.1	2.4	2.8	3.2	3.5	3.8	4.2	4.6	5.0
KILOCALORIES USED (Kcal/m)	4.5	6.0	7.5	9.0	10.5	12.0	14.0	16.0	17.5	19.0	21.0	23.0	25.0

[a] Heart rate.

FIGURE A.4. Guide to setting work loads for submaximal bicycle test

DIRECTIONS

1. Set the first work load at 300 kilopond meters per minute (1.0 kilopond).
2. If heart rate in third minute is: Less than (<) 90, set second load at 900 kilopond meters per minute (3 kilopond).
     Between 90 and 105, set second load at 750 kilopond meters per minute (2.5 kilopond).
     Greater than (>) 105, set second load at 600 kilopond meters per minute (2.0 kilopond).
3. Follow the same pattern for setting third and final load.

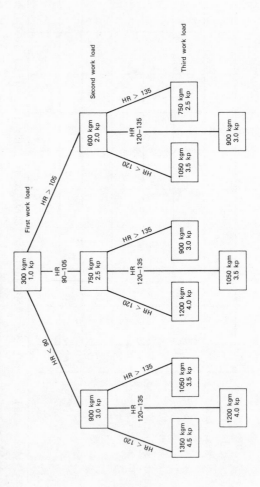

load is shown in Figure A.4. The third 3 minute work bout is counted in the same manner as the first two work periods.

The heart rate is determined by measuring the length of time it takes to count 30 heart beats. This is usually done with a stopwatch and can be measured from an ECG strip or with the use of a stethoscope. If neither is available, then one can count the pulse at the carotid artery (next to the Adam's apple). Refer to Table A.20 for ease in computing heart beats per minute. If a stopwatch is not available, the heart rate can be determined by using the second sweephand on a wrist watch and counting the heart beats for 15 seconds and multiplying by 4.

During the test the ECG information should be recorded as described under maximal stress test protocols, and blood pressure determined at the end of each three minutes of work. The recovery period is generally recorded in the supine position or pedalling on the ergometer at a very low work rate (100 to 150 kilopond meters per minute).

To estimate maximal oxygen uptake, record the final heart rate values from the second and third work bouts in accordance with the amount of work performed at each of these work loads, respectively. The first three minute work bout is not used in the calculation. Next, draw a horizontal line across the top of the form (Table A.19) corresponding to one's maximum heart rate. If maximum heart rate is not known, then it can be estimated from Table A.18. Then draw a straight line through the two heart rate values until it intersects the maximum heart rate line. The point at which the lines intersect is where the maximum oxygen uptake value is found. At this point, draw a vertical line downward to where one can read the maximum oxygen uptake in liters per minute. Finally, to express the maximum oxygen uptake in milliliters per kilogram of body weight per minute, divide the liters per minute value by body weight in kilograms (kg = lb of body weight ÷ by 2.2). To determine the participant's relative fitness level, compare the estimated value to the age adjusted norms found in Tables A.4 to A.13.

Submaximal Bench Stepping Test. The prediction of maxium oxygen uptake (or functional capacity) also can be determined by a submaximal bench stepping test. The basic assumption of this test is that, given an equal amount of work to accomplish (stepping up and down on a bench at the same rate and total time), the participant with a lower heart rate will be in better physical condition, and therefore will have a higher maximum oxygen uptake.

TABLE A.20. Conversion of the time for 30 pulse beats to pulse rate per minute

SECONDS	PER MINUTE	SECONDS	PER MINUTE	SECONDS	PER MINUTE
33.0	54	28.5	63	24.0	75
32.9	55	28.4	63	23.9	75
32.8	55	28.3	64	23.8	76
32.7	55	28.2	64	23.7	76
32.6	55	28.1	64	23.6	76
32.5	55	28.0	64	23.5	77
32.4	56	27.9	64	23.4	77
32.3	56	27.8	65	23.3	77
32.2	56	27.7	65	23.2	78
32.1	56	27.6	65	32.1	78
32.0	56	27.5	65	23.0	78
31.9	56	27.4	66	22.9	79
31.8	57	27.3	66	22.8	79
31.7	57	27.2	66	22.7	79
31.6	57	27.1	66	22.6	80
31.5	57	27.0	67	22.5	80
31.4	57	26.9	67	22.4	80
31.3	57	26.8	67	22.3	81
31.2	58	26.7	67	22.2	81
31.1	58	26.6	68	22.1	81
31.0	58	26.5	68	22.0	82
30.9	58	26.4	68	21.9	82
30.8	58	26.3	68	21.8	83
30.7	59	26.2	69	21.7	83
30.6	59	26.1	69	21.6	83
30.5	59	26.0	69	21.5	84
30.4	59	25.9	69	21.4	84
30.3	59	25.8	70	21.3	85
30.2	60	25.7	70	21.2	85
30.1	60	25.6	70	21.1	85
30.0	60	25.5	71	21.0	86
29.9	60	25.4	71	20.9	86
29.8	60	25.3	71	20.8	87
29.7	61	25.2	71	20.7	87
29.6	61	25.1	72	20.6	87
29.5	61	25.0	72	20.5	88
29.4	61	24.9	72	20.4	88
29.3	61	24.8	72	20.3	89
29.2	62	24.7	73	20.2	89
29.1	62	24.6	73	20.1	90
29.0	62	24.5	73	20.0	90
28.9	62	24.4	74	19.9	90
28.8	62	24.3	74	19.8	91
28.7	63	24.2	74	19.7	91
28.6	63	24.1	75	19.6	92

TABLE A.20. **(Continued)** Conversion of the time for 30 pulse beats rate per minute

SECONDS	PER MINUTE	SECONDS	PER MINUTE	SECONDS	PER MINUTE
19.5	92	15.0	120	10.5	171
19.4	93	14.9	121	10.4	173
19.3	93	14.8	122	10.3	175
19.2	94	14.7	122	10.2	176
19.1	94	14.6	123	10.1	178
19.0	95	14.5	124	10.0	180
18.9	95	14.4	125	9.9	182
18.8	96	14.3	126	9.8	184
18.7	96	14.2	127	9.7	186
18.6	97	14.1	128	9.6	188
18.5	97	14.0	129	9.5	189
18.4	98	13.9	129	9.4	191
18.3	98	13.8	130	9.3	194
18.2	99	13.7	131	9.2	196
18.1	99	13.6	132	9.1	198
18.0	100	13.5	133	9.0	200
17.9	101	13.4	134	8.9	202
17.8	101	13.3	135	8.8	205
17.7	102	13.2	136	8.7	207
17.6	102	13.1	137	8.6	209
17.5	103	13.0	138	8.5	212
17.4	103	12.9	140	8.4	214
17.3	104	12.8	141	8.3	217
17.2	105	12.7	142	8.2	220
17.1	105	12.6	143	8.1	222
17.0	106	12.5	144	8.0	225
16.9	107	12.4	145		
16.8	107	12.3	146		
16.7	108	12.2	148		
16.6	108	12.1	149		
16.5	109	12.0	150		
16.4	110	11.9	151		
16.3	110	11.8	153		
16.2	111	11.7	154		
16.1	112	11.6	155		
16.0	113	11.5	157		
15.9	113	11.4	158		
15.8	114	11.3	159		
15.7	115	11.2	161		
15.6	115	11.1	162		
15.5	116	11.0	164		
15.4	117	10.9	165		
15.3	118	10.8	167		
15.2	118	10.7	168		
15.1	119	10.6	170		

The test is accomplished by stepping up and down on a bench 16¼ inches high (generally the height of a bleacher seat) for a total of three minutes. Men step at a rate of 24 steps per minute, and women at 22 steps per minute. Again, it is best to use a metronome. On the completion of the three minute test, the participant remains standing while the pulse is counted for a 15-second interval, beginning 5 seconds after termination of the test. To convert the recovery heart rate to beats per minute, the 15-second heart rate is multiplied by four. The equations for estimating maximum oxygen uptake are as follows.

Men: 111.33 - (0.42 × step test pulse rate, beats/min)
Women: 65.81 - (0.1847 × step test pulse rate, beats/min)

For ease of estimating the proper value, see Table A.21. The standards shown in Table A.21 are from data collected on college age men and women; hence, information collected on middle aged participants could give slightly lower oxygen uptake values.

It would be difficult to measure blood pressure during the bench stepping test, but it should be measured as soon as possible after the 15-second, heart rate count is made. Other aspects of the exercise and recovery, that is, ECG response and heart rate, should be determined as described under maximal exercise tolerance testing.

Submaximal Testing Protocols and Field Tests to Determine Functional Capacity: Without ECG and Blood Pressure Monitoring

The submaximal exercise tolerance testing protocols recommended here are essentially the same tests as outlined under Table 3.2, Plan B, submaximal exercise tolerance testing protocols, except that the ECG and blood pressure monitoring are omitted. These tests are shown in Table 3.2, Plan C. Tests that do not monitor ECG and blood pressure should not be used for diagnostic purposes. Thus, they are used only when monitoring equipment is not available and with apparently healthy, low-risk persons under 35 years of age. They also can be used as a follow-up test for persons who have already had a diagnostic type stress test and are considered at low risk and free from heart disease.

BODY COMPOSITION

The principle of the underwater weighing technique was described in Section 3. The technique requires that a person be weighed underwater and at the same time account for the air in the lungs. Air in the lungs will make one buoyant, thus giving a spurious value. Even when one trys to blow all the air out of the lungs, there is approximately 1 to 2 liters of air that remains. This is called the residual volume. For the purposes of this book, it is assumed that the residual volume will not be measured precisely, but is estimated. It is possible in college age or younger individuals to use an assumed constant residual volume without sacrificing too much accuracy. Estimated volumes by age and sex are listed in Table A.22.

To determine body composition by underwater weighing, a scale is attached to the diving board or is hung from some other form of support, approximately 18 to 24 inches from the edge of the pool, at a point where the water is at least three feet deep. (If finances and space are available, a small pool, 4 X 4 X 5 ft., can be constructed). The scale should be accurately calibrated prior to use by hanging known weights from the scale and noting the reading. Since the residual lung volume is measured in liters, weight must also be expressed in metric units, that is, kilograms (weight in pounds divided by 2.2). See Table A.23 for conversion chart for body weight in kilograms and pounds. Individuals to be assessed sit on a chair, a weight, or some other type of seat suspended from the scale, or simply hang from a rope or chain attached to the scale. The underwater weight of individuals is determined by having them totally submerge, exhaling as they go underwater. The highest weight attained at the conclusion of their maximal exhalation represents their gross underwater weight. A minimum of 5 to 10 trials should be given each individual, since it takes practice and experience before an accurate weight can be obtained. The average of the two or three heaviest trials is selected as the representative gross weight for that individual. The weight of the seat, chair, or other supporting material must then be subtracted from the gross weight to obtain the individual's actual or net weight underwater. Body density is then calculated as follows:

$$\text{Density} = \frac{\text{body weight}}{\text{body volume}}$$

$$\text{Body volume} = \frac{(\text{weight (kg)} - \text{net underwater weight})}{\text{density of water}} - \text{estimated residual volume}$$

Since most pools are heated to approximately 76 to 78°F, a constant

TABLE A.21. Percentile rankings for recovery heart rate and predicted maximal oxygen consumption for male and female college students.

PERCENTILE RANKING	RECOVERY HR FEMALE	PREDICTED MAX VO2a (ml/kg min)	RECOVERY HR MALE	PREDICTED MAX VO2 (ml/kg min)
100	128	42.2	120	60.9
95	140	40.0	124	59.3
90	148	38.5	128	57.6
85	152	37.7	136	54.2
80	156	37.0	140	52.5
75	158	36.6	144	50.9
70	160	36.3	148	49.2
65	162	35.9	149	48.8
60	163	35.7	152	47.5
55	164	35.5	154	46.7
50	166	35.1	156	45.8
45	168	34.8	160	44.1
40	170	34.4	162	43.3
35	171	34.2	164	42.5
30	172	34.0	166	41.6
25	176	33.3	168	40.8
20	180	32.6	172	39.1
15	182	32.2	176	37.4
10	184	31.8	178	36.6
5	196	29.6	184	34.1

From F. Katch and W. McArdie. *Nutrition, Weight Control and Exercise.* Copyright 1977 by Houghton Mifflin Company. Reprinted by permission of publisher.

[a]Max $\dot{V}O_2$ = maximum oxygen uptake

Table A.22. Estimated residual volumes by sex and age

AGE (years)	ESTIMATED RESIDUAL VOLUME (liters)
Females	
6-10	0.60
11-15	0.80
16-20	1.00
21-25	1.20
26-30	1.40
Males	
6-10	0.90
11-15	1.10
16-20	1.30
21-25	1.50
26-30	1.70

TABLE A.23. Conversion Table—pounds and kilograms
(1 lb = 2.2047 kg)

POUNDS	KILO-GRAMS	POUNDS	KILO-GRAMS	POUNDS	KILO-GRAMS	POUNDS	KILO-GRAMS
100	45.36	137	62.14	174	78.92	211	95.70
101	45.81	138	62.59	175	79.38	212	96.16
102	46.26	139	63.05	176	79.83	213	96.61
103	46.72	140	63.50	177	80.28	214	97.07
104	47.17	141	63.95	178	80.74	215	97.52
105	47.63	142	64.41	179	81.19	216	97.97
106	48.08	143	64.86	180	81.64	217	98.43
107	48.53	144	65.32	181	82.10	218	98.88
108	49.00	145	65.77	182	82.55	219	99.33
109	49.44	146	66.22	183	83.00	220	99.79
110	49.89	147	66.68	184	83.46	221	100.24
111	50.35	148	67.13	185	83.91	222	100.69
112	50.80	149	67.58	186	84.37	223	101.15
113	51.25	150	68.04	187	84.82	224	101.60
114	51.71	151	68.49	188	85.27	225	102.05
115	52.16	152	68.94	189	85.73	226	102.51
116	52.61	153	69.40	190	86.18	227	102.96
117	53.07	154	69.85	191	86.63	228	103.42

TABLE A.23. (Continued) Conversion Table—pounds and kilograms

lb	kg	lb	kg	lb	kg	lb	kg
118	53.52	155	70.30	192	87.09	229	103.87
119	54.00	156	70.76	193	87.54	230	104.32
120	54.43	157	71.21	194	87.99	231	104.78
121	54.88	158	71.67	195	88.45	232	105.23
122	55.34	159	72.12	196	88.90	233	105.69
123	55.79	160	72.57	197	89.35	234	106.14
124	56.24	161	73.03	198	89.81	235	106.59
125	56.70	162	73.48	199	90.26	236	107.04
126	57.15	163	73.93	200	90.72	237	107.50
127	57.60	164	74.39	201	91.17	238	107.95
128	58.06	165	74.84	202	91.62	239	108.40
129	58.51	166	75.29	203	92.08	240	108.86
130	58.96	167	75.75	204	92.53	241	109.31
131	59.42	168	76.20	205	92.98	242	109.77
132	59.87	169	76.65	206	93.44	243	110.22
133	60.33	170	77.11	207	93.89	244	110.67
134	60.78	171	77.56	208	94.34	245	111.13
135	61.23	172	78.02	209	94.80	246	111.58
136	61.69	173	78.47	210	95.25	247	112.03
						248	112.49
						249	112.94
						250	113.39

density of water of 0.997 will be used.

$$\text{Relative fat, \%} = [(495/\text{density}) - 450]$$
$$\text{Fat weight} = \text{weight} \times \text{relative fat}/100$$
$$\text{Lean weight} = \text{weight} - \text{fat weight}$$

As an example of the above, a male who is 18 years of age weighs 180 pounds and has a net underwater weight of 8 pounds. His estimated residual volume from Table A.22 would be 1.30 liters. His body composition would be calculated as follows:

$$\text{Weight} = 180 \text{ lb} = 81.6 \text{ kg}$$
$$\text{Net underwater weight} = 8 \text{ lb} = 3.6 \text{ kg}$$

$$\text{Volume} = \frac{(81.6 - 3.6)}{0.997} - 1.3 = 78.2 - 1.3 = 76.9$$

$$\text{Density} = \frac{81.6}{76.9} = 1.061$$

$$\text{Relative fat, \%} = [(495/1.061) - 450] = 466.5 - 450 = 16.5\%$$
$$\text{Fat weight} = 16.5\% \times 180 \text{ lb}/100 = 29.7 \text{ lb}$$
$$\text{Lean weight} = 180 \text{ lb} - 29.7 = 150.3 \text{ lb}$$

Table A.24 is an example of a recording form for selected anthropometric measures (7 skinfold fat, 14 girth, and 9 diameters).

Tables A.25 to A.29 are additional conversion tables for predicting body density from anthropometric measures. Table A.25 was derived from young men; Table A.26, from young women; Table A.27, from middle-aged men; Table A.28, from middle-aged women; and, Table A.29, from world class distance runners. As mentioned in Section 3, prediction equations with a combination of skinfold, girth, and diameter measures usually give higher predictions of body density. Thus, if the equipment and time are available, the conversion tables shown in Tables A.25 to A.29 are preferred over Table 3.4 to 3.18.

TABLE A.24. Recording form for anthropometric measures.[a]

Body Composition & Pulmonary Function

INSTITUTE FOR AEROBICS RESEARCH

PATIENT NO.
B T X - |___|___| - |___|___|___|
VISIT FORM
|___| P

Name: |_____| Date: |__|/|__|/|__|
Last Name First   MONTH DAY YEAR
Age: |___| Body Wt: |_____| kg [1]   Ht: |_____| cm [1]   Bar. Pr. |_____| mm
                              lb [2]   in [2]
Group: |_____| Sex: □

SKINFOLD FAT

	Trial 1 □	Trial 2 □	DIMENSIONS	Trial 1 □	Trial 2 □
	mm	mm		cm	cm
CHEST	|___._|	|___._|	BIDELTOID	|____._____|	|____._____|
AXILLA	|___._|	|___._|	BIACROMIAL	|____._____|	|____._____|
TRICEPS	|___._|	|___._|	CHEST WIDTH	|____._____|	|____._____|
SUBSCAPULAR	|___._|	|___._|	CHEST DEPTH	|____._____|	|____._____|
ABDOMINAL	|___._|	|___._|	BICRISTAL	|____._____|	|____._____|
SUPRAILIAC	|___._|	|___._|	BITROCHANTERIC	|____._____|	|____._____|
THIGH	|___._|	|___._|	KNEE WIDTH	|___._____|	|___._____|
SUM OF 6	|_____._|	|_____._|	WRIST WIDTH	|___._____|	|___._____|
SUM OF 7	|_____._|	|_____._|	ELBOW WIDTH	|___._____|	|___._____|

GIRTH

	Trial 1 □	Trial 2 □		Trial 1 □	Trial 2 □
	cm	cm		cm	cm
SHOULDER	|_____._____|	|_____._____|	GLUTEAL	|_____._____|	|_____._____|
CHEST (N)	|_____._____|	|_____._____|	THIGH	|____._____|	|____._____|
CHEST (INF)	|_____._____|	|_____._____|	CALF	|___._____|	|___._____|
CHEST (DEF)	|_____._____|	|_____._____|	ANKLE	|___._____|	|___._____|
CHEST EXPAN.	|___._____|	|_____._____|	BICEPS	|___._____|	|___._____|
ABDOMEN	|____._____|	|____._____|	FOREARM	|___._____|	|___._____|
WAIST	|_____._____|	|_____._____|	WRIST	|___._____|	|___._____|

CUP SIZE □ BIRTH CONTROL PILLS yes [1]   DATE OF LAST PERIOD: |__|/|__|/|__|
(A=1, B=2, C=3, D=4, E=5)   no [2]   MONTH DAY YEAR

[a]Published with permission of the Institute for Aerobics Research, Dallas, Texas.

TABLE A.25. Conversion table for prediction of body fat for young men[a],[b]

SUM 7 SKINFOLD	CONVERSION FACTOR	BIACROMIAL	CONVERSION FACTOR	HEIGHT cm	HEIGHT in.	CONVERSION FACTOR
50	1.09640	30.0	04869	162	63.8	07128
52	1.09588	30.5	04950	163	64.2	07172
54	1.09536	31.0	05031	164	64.2	07216
56	1.09484	31.5	05112	165	65.0	07260
58	1.09432	32.0	05194	166	65.4	07304
60	1.09380	32.5	05275	167	65.7	07348
62	1.09328	33.0	05356	168	66.1	07392
64	1.09276	33.5	05437	169	66.5	07436
66	1.09224	34.0	05518	170	66.9	07480
68	1.09172	34.5	05599	171	67.3	07524
70	1.09120	35.0	05681	172	67.7	07568
72	1.09068	35.5	05762	173	68.1	07612
74	1.09016	36.0	05843	174	68.5	07656
76	1.08964	36.5	05924	175	68.9	07700
78	1.08912	37.0	06005	176	69.3	07744
80	1.08860	37.5	06086	177	69.7	07788
82	1.08808	38.0	06167	178	70.1	07832
84	1.08756	38.5	06249	179	70.5	07876
86	1.08704	39.0	06330	180	70.9	07920
88	1.08652	39.5	06411	181	71.3	07964
90	1.08600	40.0	06492	182	71.7	08008
92	1.08548	40.5	06573	183	72.0	08052
94	1.08496	41.0	06654	184	72.4	08096
96	1.08444	41.5	06735	185	72.8	08140
98	1.08392	42.0	06817	186	73.2	08184

YOUNG MEN[a]

PERSONAL MEASUREMENTS

Sum-7 _____cm

Biacromial _____cm

Height _____cm (in.)

CONVERSIONS

Sum-7 _____

+

Biacromial _____

—

Height _____

=

Density _____

(gm/cc)

(Density is the sum of conversion factors.)

TABLE A.25. (Continued) Conversion table for prediction of body fat for young men[a,b]

SUM 7 SKINFOLD	CONVERSION FACTOR	BIACROMIAL	CONVERSION FACTOR	HEIGHT cm	HEIGHT in.	CONVERSION FACTOR
100	1.08340	42.5	06898	187	73.6	08228
102	1.08288	43.0	06979	188	74.0	08272
104	1.08236	43.5	07060	189	74.4	08316
106	1.08184	44.0	07141	190	74.8	08360
108	1.08132	44.5	07222	191	75.2	08404
110	1.08080	45.0	07304	192	75.6	08448
112	1.08028	45.5	07385	193	76.0	08492
114	1.07976	46.0	07466	194	76.4	08536
116	1.07924	46.5	07547	195	76.8	08580
118	1.07872	47.0	07628	196	77.2	08624
120	1.07820	47.5	07709	197	77.6	08668
122	1.07768	48.0	07790	198	78.0	08712
124	1.07716	48.5	07872	199	78.3	08756
126	1.07664	49.0	07953	200	78.7	08800
128	1.07612	49.5	08034	201	79.1	08844
130	1.07560	50.0	08115	202	79.5	08888
132	1.07508	50.5	08196	203	79.9	08932
134	1.07456	51.0	80277	204	80.3	08976
136	1.07404	51.5	08358	205	80.7	09020
138	1.07352	52.0	08440	206	81.1	09064
140	1.07300	52.5	08521	207	81.5	09108
142	1.07248	53.0	08602	208	81.9	09152
144	1.08196	53.5	08683	209	82.3	09196
146	1.07144	54.0	08764	210	82.7	09244
148	1.08092	54.5	08845	211	83.1	09284
150	1.07040	55.0	08927	212	83.5	09328

[a]Table developed by M.L. Pollock (Institute for Aerobics Research) and A.J. Jackson (University of Houston).
[b]Pollock, Hickman, Kendrick, Jackson, Linnerud, and Dawson. Prediction of body density in young and middle-aged men. 40:300-304 (1976).

Density = 1.1094 − 0.00026 X sum-7 + 0.001623 X biacromial − 0.00044 X height
R = 0.87 Standard error = 0.0070

TABLE A.26. Conversion table for prediction of percent body fat for young women[a,b]

SUPRAILIAC SKINFOLD (mm)	CONVERSION FACTOR	THIGH SKINFOLD (mm)	CONVERSION FACTOR	WRIST GIRTH (mm)	CONVERSION FACTOR	KNEE DIAMETER (mm)	CONVERSION FACTOR	YOUNG WOMEN
1	1.0829	1	0.0007	5.0	0.0240	3.0	0.0264	PERSONAL MEASUREMENTS
2	1.0822	2	0.0014	5.5	0.0264	3.5	0.0308	
3	1.0815	3	0.0021	6.0	0.0288	4.0	0.0352	Suprailiac _____ mm
4	1.0808	4	0.0028	6.5	0.0312	4.5	0.0396	
5	1.0801	5	0.0035	7.0	0.0336	5.0	0.0440	Thigh _____ mm
6	1.0794	6	0.0042	7.5	0.0360	5.5	0.0484	
7	1.0787	7	0.0049	8.0	0.0384	6.0	0.0528	Wrist _____ cm
8	1.0780	8	0.0056	8.5	0.0408	6.5	0.0572	
9	1.0773	9	0.0063	9.0	0.0432	7.0	0.0616	Knee _____ cm
10	1.0766	10	0.0070	9.5	0.0456	7.5	0.0660	
11	1.0759	11	0.0077	10.0	0.0480	8.0	0.0704	CONVERSIONS
12	1.0752	12	0.0084	10.5	0.0504	8.5	0.0748	
13	1.0745	13	0.0091	11.0	0.0528	9.0	0.0792	Suprailiac _____
14	1.0738	14	0.0098	11.5	0.0552	9.5	0.0836	−
15	1.0731	15	0.0105	12.0	0.0576	10.0	0.0880	Thigh _____
16	1.0724	16	0.0112	12.5	0.0600	10.5	0.0924	+
17	1.0717	17	0.0119	13.0	0.0624	11.0	0.0968	Wrist _____
18	1.0710	18	0.0126	13.5	0.0648	11.5	0.1012	−
19	1.0703	19	0.0133	14.0	0.0672	12.0	0.1056	Knee _____
20	1.0696	20	0.0140	14.5	0.0696	12.5	0.1100	=
21	1.0689	21	0.0147	15.0	0.0720	13.0	0.1144	Density _____
22	1.0682	22	0.0154	15.5	0.0744	13.5	0.1188	(gm/cc)
23	1.0675	23	0.0161	16.0	0.0768	14.0	0.1232	(Density is the sum of
24	1.0668	24	0.0168	16.5	0.0792	14.5	0.1276	conversion factors.)
25	1.0661	25	0.0175	17.0	0.0816	15.0	0.1320	

TABLE A.26. (Continued) Conversion table for prediction of percent body fat for young women[a,b]

SUPRAILIAC SKINFOLD (mm)	CONVERSION FACTOR	THIGH SKINFOLD (mm)	CONVERSION FACTOR	WRIST GIRTH (mm)	CONVERSION FACTOR	KNEE DIAMETER (mm)	CONVERSION FACTOR
26	1.0654	26	0.0182	17.5	0.0840	15.5	0.1364
27	1.0647	27	0.0189	18.0	0.0864	16.0	0.1408
28	1.0640	28	0.0196	18.5	0.0888	16.5	0.1452
29	1.0633	29	0.0203	19.0	0.0912	17.0	0.1496
30	1.0626	30	0.0210	19.5	0.0936	17.5	0.1540
31	1.0619	31	0.0217	20.0	0.0960	18.0	0.1584
32	1.0612	32	0.0224	20.5	0.0984	18.5	0.1628
33	1.0605	33	0.0231	21.0	0.1008	19.0	0.1672
34	1.0598	34	0.0238	21.5	0.1032	19.5	0.1716
35	1.0591	35	0.0245	22.0	0.1056	20.0	0.1760
36	1.0584	36	0.0252	22.5	0.1080	20.5	0.1804
37	1.0577	37	0.0259	23.0	0.1104	21.0	0.1848
38	1.0570	38	0.0266	23.5	0.1128	21.5	0.1892
39	1.0563	39	0.0273	24.0	0.1152	22.0	0.1936
40	1.0556	40	0.0280	24.5	0.1176	22.5	0.1980
41	1.0549	41	0.0287	25.0	0.1200	23.0	0.2024
42	1.0542	42	0.0294	25.5	0.1224	23.5	0.2068
43	1.0535	43	0.0301	26.0	0.1248	24.0	0.2112
44	1.0528	44	0.0308	26.5	0.1272	24.5	0.2156
45	1.0521	45	0.0315	27.0	0.1296	25.0	0.2200
46	1.0514	46	0.0322	27.5	0.1320	25.5	0.2244
47	1.0507	47	0.0329	28.0	0.1344	26.0	0.2288
48	1.0500	48	0.0336	28.5	0.1368	26.5	0.2332
49	1.0493	49	0.0343	29.0	0.1392	27.0	0.2376
50	1.0486	50	0.0350	29.5	0.1416	27.5	0.2420

[a]Table developed by M.L. Pollock (Institute for Aerobics Research) and A.J. Jackson (University of Houston).

[b]Pollock, Laughridge, Coleman, Linnerud, and Jackson. "Prediction of body density in young and middle-aged women." *J. Appl. Physiol.,* 38:745-749 (1975).

Density = $1.0836 - 0.0007$ X suprailiac $- 0.0007$ X thigh $+ 0.0048$ X wrist $- 0.0088$ X knee

$R = 0.826$ standard error $= 0.0082$

TABLE A.27. Conversion table for prediction of percent body fat for middle-aged men[a,b]

CHEST SKINFOLD (mm)	CONVERSION FACTOR	AXILLA SKINFOLD (mm)	CONVERSION FACTOR	GLUTEAL SKINFOLD (mm)	CONVERSION FACTOR	FOREARM GIRTH (cm)	CONVERSION FACTOR
1	1.10113	1	0.00046	75	0.075	17.5	0.03973
2	1.10041	2	0.00092	76	0.076	18.0	0.04086
3	1.09969	3	0.00138	77	0.077	18.5	0.04200
4	1.09897	4	0.00184	78	0.078	19.0	0.04313
5	1.09825	5	0.00230	79	0.079	19.5	0.04427
6	1.09753	6	0.00276	80	0.080	20.0	0.04540
7	1.09681	7	0.00322	81	0.081	20.5	0.04654
8	1.09609	8	0.00368	82	0.082	21.0	0.04767
9	1.09537	9	0.00414	83	0.083	21.5	0.04881
10	1.09465	10	0.00460	84	0.084	22.0	0.04994
11	1.09393	11	0.00506	85	0.085	22.5	0.05108
12	1.09321	12	0.00552	86	0.086	23.0	0.05221
13	1.09249	13	0.00598	87	0.087	23.5	0.05335
14	1.09177	14	0.00644	88	0.088	24.0	0.05448
15	1.09105	15	0.00690	89	0.089	24.5	0.05562
16	1.09033	16	0.00736	90	0.090	25.0	0.05675
17	1.08961	17	0.00782	91	0.091	25.5	0.05789
18	1.08889	18	0.00828	92	0.092	26.0	0.05902
19	1.08817	19	0.00874	93	0.093	26.5	0.06016
20	1.08945	20	0.00920	94	0.094	27.0	0.06129
21	1.08673	21	0.00966	95	0.095	27.5	0.06243
22	1.08601	22	0.01012	96	0.096	28.0	0.06356
23	1.08529	23	0.01058	97	0.097	28.5	0.06470
24	1.08457	24	0.01104	98	0.098	29.0	0.06583
25	1.08385	25	0.01150	99	0.099	29.5	0.06697

MIDDLE-AGED MEN

PERSONAL MEASUREMENTS

Chest _____ mm

Axilla _____ mm

Gluteal _____ cm

Forearm _____ cm

CONVERSIONS

Chest _____

− Axilla _____

− Gluteal _____

+ Forearm _____

= Density (gm/cc) _____

(Density is the sum of conversion factors.)

TABLE A.27. (Continued) Conversion table for prediction of percent body fat for middle-aged men[a,b]

CHEST SKINFOLD (mm)	CONVERSION FACTOR	AXILLA SKINFOLD (mm)	CONVERSION FACTOR	GLUTEAL SKINFOLD (mm)	CONVERSION FACTOR	FOREARM GIRTH (cm)	CONVERSION FACTOR
26	1.08313	26	0.01196	100	0.100	30.0	0.06810
27	1.08241	27	0.01242	101	0.101	30.5	0.06924
28	1.08169	28	0.01288	102	0.102	31.0	0.07037
29	1.08097	29	0.01334	103	0.103	31.5	0.07151
30	1.08025	30	0.01380	104	0.104	32.0	0.07264
31	1.07953	31	0.01426	105	0.105	32.5	0.07378
32	1.07881	32	0.01472	106	0.106	33.0	0.07491
33	1.07809	33	0.01518	107	0.107	33.5	0.07605
34	1.07737	34	0.01564	108	0.108	34.0	0.07718
35	1.07665	35	0.01610	109	0.109	34.5	0.07832
36	1.07593	36	0.01656	110	0.110	35.0	0.07945
37	1.07521	37	0.01702	111	0.111	35.5	0.08059
38	1.07449	38	0.01748	112	0.112	36.0	0.08172
39	1.07377	39	0.01794	113	0.113	36.5	0.08286
40	1.07305	40	0.01840	114	0.114	37.0	0.08399
41	1.07233	41	0.01886	115	0.115	37.5	0.08513
42	1.07161	42	0.01932	116	0.116	38.0	0.08626
43	1.07089	43	0.01978	117	0.117	38.5	0.08740
44	1.07017	44	0.02024	118	0.118	39.0	0.08853
45	1.06945	45	0.02070	119	0.119	39.5	0.08967
46	1.06873	46	0.02116	120	0.120	40.0	0.09080
47	1.06801	47	0.02162	121	0.121	40.5	0.09194
48	1.06729	48	0.02208	122	0.122	41.0	0.09307
49	1.06657	49	0.02254	123	0.123	41.5	0.09421
50	1.06585	50	0.02300	124	0.124	42.0	0.09534

[a]Table developed by M.L. Pollock (Institute for Aerobics Research) and A.J. Jackson (University of Houston).

[b]Pollock, Hickman, Kendrick, Jackson, Linnerud, and Dawson. "Prediction of body density in young and middle-aged men." *40*:300-304 (1976).

Density = $1.10185 - 0.00072 \times$ chest $- 0.00046 \times$ axilla $- 0.001 \times$ gluteal $+ 0.00227 \times$ forearm

$R = 0.83$ Standard error 0.0075

TABLE A.28. Conversion table for prediction of percent body fat for middle-aged women[a,b]

SUPRAILIAC SKINFOLD (mm)	CONVERSION FACTOR	THIGH SKINFOLD (mm)	CONVERSION FACTOR	WRIST GIRTH (cm)	CONVERSION FACTOR	CUP SIZE	CONVERSION FACTOR	MIDDLE-AGED WOMEN
1	1.1018	1	0.0003	50	0.0250	0.25	0.00083	PERSONAL MEASUREMENTS
2	1.1013	2	0.0006	51	0.0255	0.50	0.00165	
3	1.1008	3	0.0009	52	0.0260	0.75	0.00248	Suprailiac ———— mm
4	1.1003	4	0.0012	53	0.0265	1.00	0.00330	
5	1.0998	5	0.0015	54	0.0270	1.25	0.00413	Thigh ———— mm
6	1.0993	6	0.0018	55	0.0275	1.50	0.00495	
7	1.0988	7	0.0021	56	0.0280	1.75	0.00578	Waist ———— cm
8	1.0983	8	0.0024	57	0.0285	2.00	0.00660	
9	1.0978	9	0.0027	58	0.0290	2.25	0.00743	Cup ———— size
10	1.0973	10	0.0030	59	0.0295	2.50	0.00825	
11	1.0968	11	0.0033	60	0.0300	2.75	0.00908	CONVERSIONS
12	1.0963	12	0.0036	61	0.0305	3.00	0.00990	
13	1.0958	13	0.0039	62	0.0310	3.25	0.01073	Suprailiac ————
14	1.0953	14	0.0042	63	0.0315	3.50	0.01155	–
15	1.0948	15	0.0045	64	0.0320	3.75	0.01238	Thigh ————
16	1.0943	16	0.0048	65	0.0325	4.00	0.01320	–
17	1.0938	17	0.0051	66	0.0330	4.25	0.01403	Waist ————
18	1.0933	18	0.0054	67	0.0335	4.50	0.01485	–
19	1.0928	19	0.0057	68	0.0340	4.75	0.01568	Cup ————
20	1.0923	20	0.0060	69	0.0345	5.00	0.01650	=
21	1.0918	21	0.0063	70	0.0350	5.25	0.01733	Density ————
22	1.0913	22	0.0066	71	0.0355	5.50	0.01815	(gm/cc)
23	1.0908	23	0.0069	72	0.0360	5.75	0.01898	(Density is the sum of
24	1.0903	24	0.0072	73	0.0365	6.00	0.01980	conversion factors.)
25	1.0890	25	0.0075	74	0.0370	6.25	0.02063	

TABLE A.28. (Continued) Conversion table for prediction of percent body fat for middle-aged women[a,b]

SUPRAILIAC SKINFOLD (mm)	CONVERSION FACTOR	THIGH SKINFOLD (mm)	CONVERSION FACTOR	WRIST GIRTH (cm)	CONVERSION FACTOR	CUP SIZE	CONVERSION FACTOR
26	1.0893	26	0.0078	75	0.0375	6.50	0.02145
27	1.0888	27	0.0081	76	0.0380	6.75	0.02228
28	1.0883	28	0.0084	77	0.0385	7.00	0.02310
29	1.0878	29	0.0087	78	0.0390		
30	1.0873	30	0.0090	79	0.0395		
31	1.0868	31	0.0093	80	0.0400		
32	1.0863	32	0.0096	81	0.0405		
33	1.0858	33	0.0099	82	0.0410		
34	1.0853	34	0.0102	83	0.0415		
35	1.0848	35	0.0105	84	0.0420		
36	1.0843	36	0.0108	85	0.0425		
37	1.0836	37	0.0111	86	0.0430		
38	1.0833	38	0.0114	87	0.0435		
39	1.0829	39	0.0117	88	0.0440		
40	1.0823	40	0.0120	89	0.0445		
41	1.0818	41	0.0123	90	0.0450		
42	1.0813	42	0.0126	91	0.0455		
43	1.0808	43	0.0129	92	0.0460		
44	1.0803	44	0.0132	93	0.0465		
45	1.0798	45	0.0135	94	0.0470		
46	1.0793	46	0.0138	95	0.0475		
47	1.0788	47	0.0141	96	0.0480		
48	1.0783	48	0.0144	97	0.0485		
49	1.0778	49	0.0147	98	0.0490		
50	1.0773	50	0.0150	99	0.0495		

[a]Table developed by M.L. Pollock (Institute for Aerobics Research) and A.J. Jackson (University of Houston).
[b]Pollock, Laughridge, Coleman, Linnerud, and Jackson. "Prediction of body density in young and middle-aged women." *J. Appl. Physiol.*, 38:745-749 (1975).

Density = $1.1023 - 0.0005 \times$ supprailiac $- 0.0003 \times$ thigh $- 0.0005 \times$ waist $- 0.0033 \times$ cup
$R = 0.889$ Standard error = 0.0069

TABLE A.29. Conversion table for prediction of percent body fat for lean males[a,b]

THIGH SKINFOLD (mm)	CONVERSION FACTOR	BIDELTOID (cm)	CONVERSION FACTOR	LEAN MALES
				PERSONAL MEASUREMENTS
1.0	1.0530	32.5	0.0390	
1.5	1.0513	33.0	0.0396	Thigh _____ mm
2.0	1.0496	33.5	0.0402	
2.5	1.0479	34.0	0.0408	Bideltoid _____ cm
3.0	1.0462	34.5	0.0414	
3.5	1.0445	35.0	0.0420	
4.0	1.0428	35.5	0.0426	CONVERSIONS
4.5	1.0411	36.0	0.0432	
5.0	1.0394	36.5	0.0438	Thigh _____
5.5	1.0377	37.0	0.0444	+
6.0	1.0360	37.5	0.0450	Bideltoid _____
6.5	1.0343	38.0	0.0456	=
7.0	1.0326	38.5	0.0462	Density _____
7.5	1.0309	39.0	0.0468	(gm/cc)
8.0	1.0292	39.5	0.0474	(Density is the sum of
8.5	1.0275	40.0	0.0480	conversion factors.)
9.0	1.0258	40.5	0.0486	
9.5	1.0241	41.0	0.0492	
10.0	1.0224	41.5	0.0498	
10.5	1.0207	42.0	0.0504	
11.0	1.0190	42.5	0.0510	
11.5	1.0173	43.0	0.0516	
12.0	1.0156	43.5	0.0522	
12.5	1.0139	44.0	0.0528	
13.0	1.0122	44.5	0.0534	

TABLE A.29. (Continued) Conversion table for prediction of percent body fat for lean males[a,b]

THIGH SKINFOLD (mm)	CONVERSION FACTOR	BIDELTOID (cm)	CONVERSION FACTOR
13.5	1.0105	45.0	0.0540
14.0	1.0088	45.5	0.0546
14.5	1.0071	46.0	0.0552
15.0	1.0054	46.5	0.0558
15.5	1.0037	47.0	0.0564
16.0	1.0020	47.5	0.0570
16.5	1.0003	48.0	0.0576
17.0	0.9986	48.5	0.0582
17.5	0.9969	49.0	0.0588
18.0	0.9952	49.5	0.0594
18.5	0.9935	50.0	0.0600
19.0	0.9918	50.5	0.0606
19.5	0.9901	51.0	0.0612
20.0	0.9884	51.5	0.0618
20.5	0.9867	52.0	0.0624
21.0	0.9850	52.5	0.0630
21.5	0.9833	53.0	0.0636
22.0	0.9816	53.5	0.0642
22.5	0.9799	54.0	0.0648
23.0	0.9782	54.5	0.0654
23.5	0.9765	55.0	0.0660
24.0	0.9748	55.5	0.0666
24.5	0.9731	56.0	0.0672
25.0	0.9714	56.5	0.0678

[a]Table developed by M.L. Pollock (Institute for Aerobics Research) and A.J. Jackson (University of Houston).
[b]Pollock, Ayres, Ward, Jackson, Linnerud, and Gettman. "Body Composition of Elite Class Distance Runners." *Ann. NY Acad. Sci.* 301:361-370 (1977).

Density = $1.0564 - 0.0034 \times$ thigh + $0.0012 \times$ bideltoid

$R = 0.87$ Standard error = 0.0038

Appendix B

American College of Sports Medicine Position Statement on "Prevention of Heat Injuries During Distance Running"

PREVENTION OF HEAT INJURIES DURING DISTANCE RUNNING*
Based on research findings and current rules governing distance running competition, it is the position of the American College of Sports Medicine that:

1. *Distance races (> 16 km or 10 miles) should not be conducted when the wet bulb temperature–globe temperature** exceeds 28° C (82.4° F).*
2. *During periods of the year, when the daylight dry bulb temperature often exceeds 27° C (80° F), distance races should be conducted before 9:00 A.M. or after 4:00 P.M.*
3. *It is the responsibility of the race sponsors to provide fluids which contain small amounts of sugar (less than 2.5 g glucose per 100 ml of water) and electrolytes (less than 10 mEq sodium and 5 mEq potassium per liter of solution.)*

4. *Runners should be encouraged to frequently ingest fluids during competition and to consume 400-500 ml (13-17 oz.) of fluid 10-15 minutes before competition.*

5. *Rules prohibiting the administration of fluids during the first 10 kilometers (6.2 miles) of a marathon race should be amended to permit fluid ingestion at frequent intervals along the race course. In light of the high sweat rates and body temperatures during distance running in the heat, race sponsors should provide "water stations" at 3-4 kilometer (2-2.5 mile) intervals for all races of 16 kilometers (10 miles) or more.*

6. *Runners should be instructed in how to recognize the early warning symptoms that precede heat injury. Recognition of symptoms, cessation of running, and proper treatment can prevent heat injury. Early warning symptoms include the following: piloerection on chest and upper arms, chilling, throbing pressure in the head, unsteadiness, nausea, and dry skin.*

7. *Race sponsors should make prior arrangements with medical personnel for the care of cases of heat injury. Responsible and informed personnel should supervise each "feeding station." Organizational personnel should reserve the right to stop runners who exhibit clear signs of heat stroke or heat exhaustion.*

It is the position of the American College of Sports Medicine that policies established by local, national, and international sponsors of distance running events should adhere to these guidelines. Failure, to adhere to these guidelines may jeopardize the health of competitors through heat injury.

*Position statement of the American College of Sports Medicine that appeared in *Medicine and Science in Sports,* Vol. 7, No. 1, 1975.

**Adapted from D. Minard, "Prevention of Heat Casualties in Marine Corps Recruits." *Milit. Med., 126*:261 (1961). WB-GT = 0.7 (WBT) + 0.2 (GT) + 0.1 (DBT).

Appendix C

Special Information Concerning Cardiac Rehabilitation

OTHER CARDIOVASCULAR DISEASES

PULMONARY HYPERTENSION High blood pressure in the circulation to the lungs can result from many causes. With these patients, unfortunately, there is often a contraindication for high-level exercise. This does not imply, however, that a patient with high pulmonary vascular resistance and hypertension from emphysema should not undertake a slowly progressing walking program. After a low-level conditioning program, the beneficial effects on peripheral distribution and blood return can be significant. One- to three-minute intervals of light exercise (walking interspersed with rest) may be particularly useful for those patients whose airways cannot conduct air rapidly but who have good circulatory reserves requiring the stimulus of activity.

ASYMMETRIC SEPTAL HYPERTROPHY (ASH) This disorder, which used to be called "idiopathic hypertrophic subaortic stenosis" is an unusual condition that often benefits from Beta blockers such as propanolol. The overthickened (hypertrophied) muscle in the left ventricle (particularly the interventricular septum) tends to block the normal flow of blood to the aorta when the left ventricle contracts. This condition is identified by a typical systolic heart murmur and by the character of the pulse on an isometric hand grip.

With ASH, exercise may aggravate the hypertrophy and produce a lack of good cardiac output leading to chest discomfort, light-headedness and actual fainting. With close medical management and follow-up, moderate, noncompetitive, endurance type exercise without isometrics is often possible. In particular, rhythym disturbances require careful individual evaluation—often using "Holter" monitoring as well as exercise tolerance testing.

ATRIOVENTRICULAR HEART BLOCK With this condition, electrical impulses originating in the atria do not get through to stimulate the fibers leading to the ventricles. Thus, the atrial contractions are out of phase with many of the slower ventricular contractions. Therefore, some cardiac efficiency is lost. Far more significant is the frequent lack of appropriate increase in ventricular rate with exercise. As a result, the requirement for increased oxygen delivery to the tissues must be accomplished by greater than usual increases in both stroke volume and arteriovenous oxygen extraction.

When heart block is discovered in the adult, it is important to have a comprehensive evaluation of the patient's status. Some individuals are born with heart block of this type and have no other reason for restricted activity. Some acquire it with infections that do not otherwise limit heart action, and some develop heart block secondarily to coronary or other diseases. This last combination may make exercise particularly hazardous. In many cases, however, an implanted electronic pacemaker can speed up the ventricular rate. Some can even be adjusted for a temporarily higher exercising pace. This is clearly an example of the great benefits derived from the taxpayers' and Heart Association contributors' support of basic and applied research.

MITRAL VALVE PROLAPSE (CLICK-MURMUR SYNDROME)
This condition, occurring most frequently in women, is relatively

newly recognized in clinical practice. It consists of a stretching of the mitral valve leaflets and their suspensory cords, leading to mitral insufficiency or regurgitation: the partial leaking of blood back into the left atrium at the time of left ventricular contraction. The prolapse that permits regurgitation usually occurs late in the left ventricular contraction time and produces a characteristically late "crescendo" murmur. Some interesting "clicks" are often heard during systole, the mechanism of which is unclear.

The more care that is taken in listening to the heart, the more cases of mitral valve prolapse show up. Echocardiography (sound signal scanning-like sonar) is a key diagnostic tool in this syndrome.

In relation to exercise, many click-murmur patients have more than their share of sharp chest pains, ventricular premature beats, and a slightly increased tendency to infections in the mitral valve. The chest pains must be differentiated from angina, and the premature beats should be evaluated relative to their hazard. Exercise testing can be helpful in both these areas. The exercise test may be abnormal, however, with ST-segment displacement early in the test, and often with hyperventilation. Frequently, there is little increase in abnormality as the heart rate, blood pressure, and "double product" increase with more demanding work. At this time it would appear unwarranted to restrict those with uncomplicated mitral valve prolapse from enjoyable, endurance stimulating activities of a moderate level—perhaps up to 10 METS. Social dancing, tennis, bicycling, swimming, skating, skiing, and jogging all seem reasonable activities, but more data are needed. It is conceivable that more vigorous activities, particularly those with an isometric component, could accelerate the stretching of the valve structures or precipitate hazardous dysrhythmias. Propanolol in mild dosages appears to help reduce both the dysrhythmia and the chest pain. This will probably reduce the tension on the valve structures as well.

It is important to indicate that some physical activities increase the probability of getting scratches and scrapes that permit bacteria to enter the circulation. Physicians, patients, coaches, family, and friends must help emphasize the need for prophylactic antibiotics to prevent infection in, on, and around the affected valves.

CASE STUDIES

Case I:

REHABILILITATION OF A PATIENT WITH MYOCARDIAL INFARCTION

Actual case reports of rehabilitation might illustrate the good results that can be obtained with patient cooperation.

"Henry" (not his real name) had a treadmill test at age 37 on 5 May, 1975. The evaluation was indicated because previously he had an elevated serum cholesterol disturbance of the Type II variety (a lipo-protein measurement category associated with high risk of coronary disease), and because his father died of a third infarct at age 43. He was an avid bicycle commuter who had reduced his cholesterol level through strict adherence to the recommended food selection. His exercise test showed a 10-MET limit with a maximum heart rate of 196.

At his age, a "normal" capacity of 12 to 13 METS might have been expected, especially with his usual 10-mile, 4-times-per-week bicycle riding and his lean, muscular build. (He probably would have shown a relatively more outstanding performance on a bicycle ergometer be-cause of his specific training in that activity). The only abnormalities noted were six consecutive sequences of two normal electrocardio-graphic complexes followed by a premature ventricular complex in the first minute of the most demanding three-minute work load. No further irregularities developed until a few ventricular prematures occurred immediately upon lying down after the treadmill was stopped. (This permits physical examination after exercise, including listening to the heart sounds. Under normal circumstances, exercise should be tapered off gradually). At no time did he have typical "ischemic-type" electrocardiographic changes so often found with developing coronary disease. He was encouraged to continue his activity and nutritional programs.

One year and three weeks later, however, he developed intermittent but impressive, often exertion-related, chest discomfort. His sweaty grey appearance and ischemic electrocardiogram prompted hospitaliza-tion in a coronary care unit. An anterior myocardial infarction was confirmed by enzyme tests and electrocardiographic changes. His frequent ventricular premature complexes were well controlled by

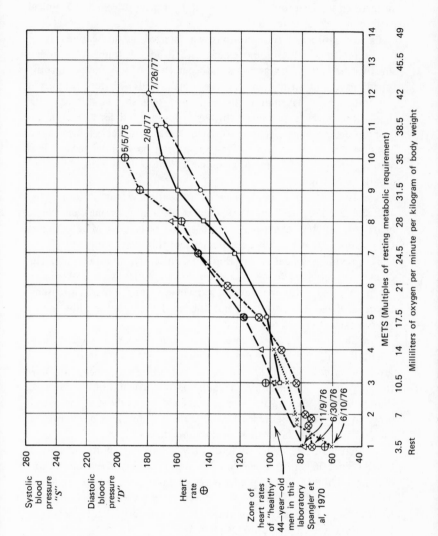

Systolic blood pressure "S"

Diastolic blood pressure "D"

Heart rate ⊕

Zone of heart rates of "healthy" 44—year—old men in this laboratory Spangler et al, 1970

METS (Multiples of resting metabolic requirement)

Milliliters of oxygen per minute per kilogram of body weight

Rest

5/5/75

2/8/77

7/26/77

11/9/76

6/30/76

6/10/76

an intravenous infusion of lidocaine, and the pain subsided in a typical pattern over the first few days.

Passive and active foot motions were started on the second day of his hospitalization. Arm movement and deep breathing were added shortly thereafter. Intravenous lidocaine was discontinued on the fourth day, and sitting on the edge of the bed with feet supported was initiated for 10 minutes twice daily. Progressive ambulation with flexibility exercises proceded through four defined levels of the in hospital protocol (See Table 5.3). After the second week, he was walking slowly in the hall while being monitored on radiotelemetry. Premature complexes were so infrequent that a long term, "Holter" monitor was not used.

On 10 June a low level treadmill evaluation was undertaken (1½, 1¾, and 2 miles per hour at 0, then at 3½ and 7% grade), eliciting a heart rate of 100 beats per minute at the peak of 4 METS (Figure C.1). Upon discharge, an exercise prescription was composed (Table C.1), providing guidance on the type, intensity, duration, and frequency of activities to be allowed. Some activities were *pro*scribed—lifting, pushing, push-ups, and auto travel—except for medical reasons. Sexual activity was permitted but the need for a mature, low energy approach was explicitly discussed.

Walking was defined in three ways: rate of work, or *speed,* with orientation during the treadmill evaluation, *heart rate* response, and level of *subjective discomfort.* Since perceptions of speed are hard to carry from a laboratory treadmill onto a neighborhood sidewalk, the "pulse rate prescription" became the chief ingredient of the overall program for this patient. He had experienced no chest discomfort in the 10 days before the exercise evaluation and discharge.

In Henry's case, an upper limit of 96 beats per minute was established. Since he did not develop (or admit to) any chest discomfort or pain on the low level, predischarge evaluation, he was restricted to no more than a Grade 1 discomfort level on a scale of 0 to 4, and told to stop activity if any palpitations or rhythm disturbance occurred. Walking was the chief exertional activity.

After the 6-MET test of 30 June (five weeks postinfarct) again without symptoms or dysrhythmia, Henry was permitted to return to his sedentary desk job (Table C.2). On hot days he was allowed to enjoy floating around in a neighborhood swimming pool with his children, but with no strokes requiring lifting his arms out of the water. Walking was still the major focus of activity. Automobile driving was permitted during noncongested hours with the understanding that he would not change tires nor carry clumsy, heavy packages. Later, he was informed how to pause between small segments of the tire changing procedure. Minor alterations and "midcourse corrections" were made over the phone or at office visits during the summer and fall.

On 9 November, 1976, approximately six months postinfarct, Henry achieved 8 METS with a maximum heart rate of 162 (Figure C.1). His final exercise prescription is provided in Table C.3 and includes bicycle riding, dancing, and most activities of daily living except snow shovelling. Jogging and noncontinuous rope skipping also would have been permitted if he had so desired, but he preferred rapid walking.

Skipping rope continuously has been shown to involve around 12 METS; he was advised to jump no more than five times in a row and then walk around while "catching his breath" before starting another sequence of five.

Had jogging been included (he did not care for it), we would have had him try a slow, electrocardiographically monitored jog on the treadmill. We would have demonstrated the importance of placing the heel down first and rolling forward to push off from the ball of the foot.

Initially there was little expansion of Henry's heart rate upper limit, although activities were of greater intensity and duration and the frequency was kept high. This must be explained to the patient along with a continuing education program. We often recommend that a walk or bicycle ride closely precede the noon or evening meal, since this tends to inhibit the hunger pangs and old appetite patterns that may lead to excessive food intake. It also tends to lighten a patient's mood, which helps support the morale of the whole family.

Our patient Henry looked in on a supervised program but opted for independent efforts that were pursued without evidence of dysrhythmia or other exercise related problems. With no apparent relation to his exercise, in September 76 he developed an inflammatory reaction in the pericardium, or lining around his heart. This caused a temporary complete stop in his physical activities, requiring bed rest and continuous aspirin (anti-inflammatory) therapy. His November 1976 test demonstrated a return to good progress, and he was given a modified version of Dr. Bruno Balke's Activity Table (Table C.4). Having achieved 8 METS, a red line was drawn indicating he was not to push beyond the 6-MET level and a green line to suggest he start at a more modest 5-MET intensity. This, coupled with the 124 beats per minute heart rate maximum (Table C.3) served as guides over the winter until his evaluation of 2 February, 1977. On this occasion he completed 11 METS (3.4 miles per hour at 16% grade) with a peak heart rate of 186 and no evidence of ischemic heart muscle (Figure C.1). This was one MET further than his preinfarct performance of 10 METS with 196 beats per minute on 5 May, 1975. On 26 July 1977, he completed three minutes at final stage of 12 METS with no ST displacement and a peak heart rate of 180 (Figure C.1).

Regrettably, we cannot guarantee such excellent progress and end results for all patients, but Henry's story is living testimony to what a person can do if he or she makes the commitment. We of the heart health team need to provide the encouragement, guidance, and protection in a manner that supports the individual in his or her successful quest for a renewal of meaningful living.

TABLE C.1. Cardiology exercise laboratory[a]   Date _6/10/76_

Tel. (202) 625-2001

Name _Henry Baker_   Date of Birth ___ Age _38_

Address _2210 W. Moore St._   Telephone ( )_____

Bethesda, Md.   Referring Physician _S. Fox_

Reason for Prescription _Initiating home exercises for postinfarct_

Period Covered by Prescription _June 11· to June 30, 1976_

1. *Type(s) of Activity Recommended*   2. *Intensity and Limits*

Walking   After a _5_-min warm-up at _1½_ mph (mile in _40_ min)
Walk at _1¾_ mph (mile in _34_ min)—slower if uphill.
Modify for cold, hot, or humid weather and with anxiety.
Reduce speed if more than grade _1+_ chest discomfort/pain
on a scale of 0 to 4 or a heart rate above _96_ /min (_24_ /15 sec).
Slow down or sit down if unusual palpitations, irregular
heart action, or dizziness occurs.

Taper off with a _5_ min cool-down at _1½_ mph.

Avoid sudden stops; if necessary, shift weight from one leg to the other to pump blood back up to the heart.

Stair Climbing   Encouraged; but not more than _1_ flight continuously and never at a rate that produces dizziness or makes a conversation difficult.

Sexual Activity—permitted with "mature," low-energy approach with orchestration of Chopin/Debussy rather than Wagner.

Level IV exercises as outlined.

Acticities *NOT* recommended at this time: _Lifting, any pushups, auto travel, except moderate static pushing/straining_

3. *Duration*

A. Warm-up _5_ min   Total walk to start at not over _15_ min

B. Active "workout" _5_ min, but not exceeding that producing a "pleasant sense of fatigue," with minimal carry-over to the next morning.

C. Cool-down _5_ min

D. Shower or bath should be neither hot nor cold as both can produce inappropriate heart action.

4. Frequency   _2 per day_

At least _5_ times per week and preferably _6 or 7_.

GENERAL RECOMMENDATIONS: _Repeat evaluation 9:30 a.m. June 30, 1976_.

Do not be competitive, even with yourself.

If you feel ill from conditions such as influenza or for any other reason, do not exercise until you have fully recovered.

_____ _J. M. Fox_ , M.D.

[a]Georgetown University Hospital, 3800 Reservoir Road, N.W. Washington, D.C. 20007

TABLE C.2. Cardiology exercise laboratory[a]   Date _6/30/76_

Name _Henry Baker_   Date of Birth _____ Age _38_____

Address _2210 W. Moore St._ Telephone (202) ___625-2001___
Bethesda, MD.

                   Referring Physician ____S. Fox____

Reason for Prescription _5 wk post anterior M.I. "uncomplicated"_

Period Covered by Prescription ___July, 1976___

1. Type(s) of Activity Recommended   2. Intensity and Limits

Walking   After a _5_ min warm-up at _1½_ mph (mile in _40_ min)
            Walk at _2_ mph (mile in _30_ min)—slower if uphill.
            Modify for cold, hot, or humid weather and with anxiety.
            Reduce speed if more than grade _1_ chest discomfort/pain
            on a scale of 0 to 4 or a heart rate above _100_ /min (_25_ /15 sec).
            Slow down or sit down if unusual palpitations, irregular
            heart action, or dizziness occurs.
            Taper off with a _5_ -min cool-down at _1½_ mph.
            Avoid sudden stops; if necessary, shift weight from one
            leg to the other to pump blood back up to the heart.

Stair   Encouraged; but not more than _1_ flight continuously and
Climbing   never at a rate that produces dizziness or makes a conversa-
            tion difficult.

Swimming   _Pool walking and elementary back stroke or arms-in-_
            water breast stroke.
            Brief swimming —not for exercise as primary
            activity.
            Bent-knee sit-ups (not more than 5 at a time).

            Activities NOT recommended at this time: _Lifting_
         more than 15 lb., pushing, pushups, straining
         (at stool, etc.).

3. *Duration* Total 20 min walking.

   A. Warm-up *5* minutes
   B. Active "workout" *10* min but not exceeding that producing a "pleasant sense of fatigue," with minimal carry-over to the next morning.
   C. Cool-down *5* min
   D. Shower or bath should be neither hot nor cold as both can produce inappropriate heart action.

4. *Frequency* *2* per day.

   At least *5* times per week and preferably *6 or 7*.

   Repeat evaluation Nov. 9, 1976. Return
GENERAL RECOMMENDATIONS: *to work 9:30 a.m. to 12:30 p.m. or less*
starting July 12, 1976.
Do not be competitive, even with yourself.
If you feel ill from conditions such as influenza or any other reason, do not exercise until you have fully recovered.

_____ *S. M. Fox* _____ ,M.D.

[a]Georgetown University Hospital, 3800 Reservoir Rd., N.W. Washington, D.C. 20007.

TABLE C.3. Cardiology exercise laboratory[a]   Date *Nov. 9, 1976*

Name *Henry Baker* Date of Birth _____ Age *38*

Address *2210 W. Moore St.* Telephone (202) *625-2001*

Bethesda, MD. _____ Referring Physician *S. M. Fox*

Reason for Prescription *6 month post M.I. rehab. update*

Period Covered by Prescription *Nov. to Dec. 1976*

1. Type(s) of Activity Recommended   *2. Intensity and Limits*

Walking _____   After a _*5*_-min warm-up at _*2*_ mph (mile in
_____ _*30*_ min) Walk at no more than _*3*_ mph (mile in
_*20*_ min)—*slower if uphill.*
Modify for cold, hot or humid weather and with
anxiety. Reduce speed if more than grade
chest discomfort/pain on a scale of 0 to 4 or a
heart rate above_*124*_/min (_*31*_/15 sec).
Slow down and stop if unusual palpitations,
irregular heart action, or dizziness.

"Social (as contrasted with competitive)
doubles and singles with "mature phil-
Table Tennis   osophy." A deliberately conservative
Badminton   warm-up is necessary, and attempts to
Tennis   modify first tennis serve to obtain ¾ speed
Paddleball   will help avoid overexertion. Not to exceed
Volleyball   grade _*1+*_ discomfort or heart rate_*124*_.
Jogging   After a _*5*_ min warm-up ar _*3*_ mph (mile in
min) walking. Jog at no more than _*4*_ mph (mile
in _*15*_ min)— slower if uphill.
Modify for cold, hot, or humid weather and
with anxiety.
Reduce speed if more than grade _*1+*_ chest dis-
comfort/pain on a scale of 0 to 4 or a heart
rate above_*124*_/min (_*31*_/15 sec).
Slow down and sit or lie if unusual palpitations,
irregular heart action, or dizziness occurs.
Taper off with a _*5*_ min cool-down at_*3*_ mph
walking.
Avoid sudden stops; if necessary, shift weight
from one leg to the other to pump blood back
up the heart.

Activities *NOT* recommended at this time:
Lifting over 24 lbs – less if clumsy, carrying
heavy, clumsy packages, pushups, snow shoveling.

3. *Duration*
   A. Warm-up _5_ min
   B. Active "workout" _20-30_ min but not exceeding that producing a "pleasant sense of fatigue," with minimal carry-over to the next morning.
   C. Cool-down _5_ min
   D. Shower or bath should be neither hot nor cold, since both can produce inappropriate heart action.
4. *Frequency* _2_ per day.

At least _5_ times per week and preferably _6 or 7_ .

GENERAL RECOMMENDATIONS: *Repeat evaluation Feb. 1977*

Do not be competitive, even with yourself.
If you feel ill from conditions such as influenza or any other reason, do not exercise until you have fully recovered.

_____ *S. M. Fox* , M.D.

[a]Georgetown University Hospital, 3800 Reservoir Rd., N.W. Washington, D.C. 20007.

TABLE C.4. Metabolic multiples (METS) required by various activities[a,b]

Activity METS	3	4	5	6	7	8	9	10	11	12
Table tennis	x	x	Increasing demands with increasing skill and duration of rallies							
Golf		Pull cart	Carry clubs							
Badminton		x	x	As with table tennis						
Volleyball		x	x	x	x	x	As above			
Tennis		Social doubles	Social doubles	Singles		Competitive				
Squash and Handball				x	x	x	Competitive			
Walking (speed in miles per hour)	3	3½	4							
Walking/Jogging		x	x	x						
Jogging/Running (miles per hour)				5	5½	6	7	8	9	
Skating			x	x	x	x	x	x		
Rope skipping					x	x	x	x	x	x
Skiing—cross country			x	x^c	x^c	x^d	x^c	x^c	x^d	x^d
Mountain hiking			x	x	x	x	x	x		
Horseback riding		x	Trot	x	Gallop					
Calisthenics, games, etc.		x	x	x	x	x				
Dynamic weight lifting / Water skiing			Disproportionate blood pressure rise may add to hazards.							
Dancing	x	x	x	x	x	x	x	x		
Cycling (speed in miles per hour)	4	6	8	10	12	13	14	15		
Rowing		x	x	x	x	x	x	x	x	x
Swimming	x	x	x	x	x	x	Competitive			

[a]Adapted by S.M. Fox, M.D. from the table of Dr. Bruno Balke, and Aspen Health Center, Aspen, Co.
[b]All intensities increase with commitment or competitiveness of approach.

[c]Intermittent
[d]Continuous

CASE II: A SLOW PROGRESSION FROM SEVERE CARDIAC INSUFFICIENCY

"Bob" (not his real name), a program producer of TV, radio, and movie series reported he "felt lousy" from tiredness, malaise, and near to occasionally active nausea for two months before a very large and disabling anterior myocardial infarction in September of 1975. At no time was he aware of discrete chest discomfort and he denied effort or emotion induced distress. For six months he had complained to his physician about belching and gastric pain but no ulcers or gastro-intestinal dyskinesia were demonstrated.

About midnight on a Saturday, when he had felt so "totally beat" that he had forgone his usual dinner out, he woke up and knew he was in "deep trouble" with chest pain deep behind the left side of the sternum (breastbone). There was no nausea or vomiting but he was in an unusual sweat (diaphoresis) that became cold and clammy as the pain spread to radiate down the left arm.

He had been a heavy cigarette smoker (80 pack-years) with no known elevation of blood pressure, cholesterol, or blood sugar. The family history contained no premature heart disease. For seven years he had been intermittently depressed, with some psychotherapy having been of use over numerous episodes. He was separted from his wife but on amicable terms.

He was admitted to the hospital with evidence of pulmonary edema (fluid in the airspaces of the lower half of the lobes of the lungs) resulting from acute inadequacy of the left ventricle as a pump. It is alleged that he was defibrillated 94 times after which a count was not kept. Most of these episodes were ventricular fibrillation, which would have been fatal if not electrically converted. It took over 16 hours to obtain relief by either finding the right therapeutic dose of lidocaine or having the irritability diminish so that control was possible.

Upon discharge to home bed rest after four weeks of hospitalization, his circulatory capacity was marginal at best. He was not evaluated relative to exertional capacity until the end of April 1976—over six months after hospital discharge. Fortunately, his formerly estranged wife had agreed to shop and cook dinner for them both, and he put together a little something for his own breakfast and lunch. He was still on sick leave from his job and almost bedridden when first evaluated. Perhaps the most encouraging event was his successful cessation of smoking in March 1976.

His blood pressure was 110/ 60, pulse 64 while supine and 106/54 and 62 beats/min while standing. Loud atrial (S_4) and ventricular (S_3) gallop sounds were heard, and the soft first heart tones suggested a slow pressure rise. The lack of usual anterior electrocardiographic forces (QS waves in V_1-V_5, small R, shallow S in V_6 and inverted T waves V_1-V_6) all indicated massive anterior left ventricular muscle damage. Although on Quinidine he still had premature ventricular complexes every 6 to 10 beats. These became much more frequent with walking exercise and he had one "couplet" (two in a row).

Exercise was initiated at 2.0 miles per hour on the horizontal treadmill. After the blood pressure slid from 120/64 to 95/65 (heart rate 68) the speed was reduced to 1.7 miles per hour. Pressure stabilized but he felt a "twinge" of discomfort. After a total of 14 minutes of slow walking he was found to have a loud quadruple rhythm—accentuated S_3 particularly and an S_4 almost as loud as his first heart tones. There were no sounds (rales) of moisture in the lungs, however. Because he was on Digoxin, it was not possible to detect if any further ischemia was produced.

From this level of severely depressed heart function he started a 10-minute, three-times-a-day, slow walking program not to produce discomfort nor dyspnea and not to increase his heart rate over 80 nor premature beats more frequent than an average of one every four beats. Initially, much of this was done in the corridors of his apartment building. Flexibility exercises, with minimal muscle force involved, were also included.

He was reassessed almost weekly with the treadmill speed slowly increased from 1.7 to 2.0 miles per hour. By July of 1976 he could tolerate 10 minutes at 2.0 miles per hour after 7 minutes warm-up at 1.7 miles per hour with only Grade I (scale 0-4) chest discomfort and only minimal circumoral pallor. In September he was tolerating brief (three minute) increments of 3½% and 7% grade with a heart rate in the high 80s. He was walking one mile a day at a slower pace. In October he was tolerating four to five minutes at 2½ miles per hour and 7½ percent grade after 16 minutes of progressive warm-up at lesser loads and was showing much greater interest in life. He sensed a new eagerness to take his one-and-one-half to two- mile daily walks at a slower pace but including some inclines of less than 6 percent. Three-miles-an-hour walking and rowing machine exercises (heart rate not over 94 with 6 rowing strokes per minute against low resistance) were instituted in November with noticeably fewer premature beats occurring both in the laboratory and when counting on his own. At .the end of 1976 he was achieving 6 METS (3.0 miles per hour, 7½% grade) after a progressive warm-up of three minutes at 2, 3, 4 and 5 METS with a maximum heart rate of 130 to 136 and blood pressures of 168/68-54. He would get winded at 3.4 miles per hour at 6 percent grade but much less than when he first started at less than 2.0 miles per hour on the horizontal.

He retired from his office job and became essentially self sufficient over the winter of 1976 to 1977, doing his own shopping and light housekeeping. He was instructed on how to break into brief efforts, the successive stages of changing an auto tire and became able to drive into the country for a day with acceptable low fatigue. Choosing not to join an exercise group when he achieved 5 METS, he probably has not progressed as rapidly as he might have. He contemplates spending the winter in the south of France and, as of September 1977, was starting four rounds of jogging for 12 left-foot plants interspersed with at least an equivalent number of cycles walking. It is contemplated that he will work upward in duration but not to exceed 50 left-foot cycles at the last of the four rounds to be undertaken daily in good weather. A sequence of 20, 30, 40, and 50 cycles is a distant goal, and only on the flat in temperate weather. Some might argue that permitting a man with loud atrial and ventricular gallops to jog briefly is not wise, particularly when these undesirable tones are accentuated after exercise. We are not aware, however, of data that truly illuminate this question.

Although cardiac enlargement persists, there were no large complete "cold spot" defects suggesting a discrete ventricular aneurysm on a Thallium isotopic postexercise myocardial perfusion scan. This study suggested small areas of exercise inducible ischemia but no marked deficits that became significantly more normal on follow-up scanning were noted after two or more hours of postexertional rest. A coronary angiographic study might be helpful in evaluating surgical opportunities but he has declined such action as long as he is expanding his capabilities. He is almost free of premature beats at either rest or exertion. As he has improved, it is most encouraging to hear the Korotkoff tones all the way down to where there is no pressure in the cuff at 5 METS or more.

Multigated isotopic blood pool ventricular wall motion studies are contemplated in the future and may be of assistance in evaluating exercise induced ventricular dysfunction. It is not known, however, how they will provide data concerning the advisability of various levels of future exercise intensity, frequency, or duration.

This case is presented to indicate that even those persons with almost no reserve capacity can make significant progress on a slowly progressive program if they are well motivated and well supported.

CASE III: PERIPHERAL ARTERIAL INSUFFICIENCY OF THE HIP, THIGH, AND LOWER LEG.

John (not his real name) was a retired military officer with crampy, right calf discomfort on uphill walking becoming more prominent as he progressed through his middle-fifties. He cut out tennis and even reduced his golf playing with a not too rapidly moving foursome using an electric cart. He became progressively more troubled by impotence until his only erections were in the early morning (3:00 to 6:00 AM) when he felt reluctant to disturb his wife. In the winter of 1974 to 1975 he found he became hypertensive on minor exertion and could walk less than a city block at about 2 miles per hour without suffering Grade 3 (scale of 0-4) crampy leg pain that was very slow to subside unless he went indoors and sat down.

Although not spilling urinary sugar, he was clearly a chemical, non-insulin requiring diabetic with an abnormal glucose tolerance. His blood pressure seldom slipped below 96 diastolic and often was over 104 until a moderately vigorous treatment program was instituted. Chest discomfort, which had been only minimal on hill climbing in the summer, was no longer elicited because of his progressive limitation of walking and intercourse. He did little manual work with his hands as a manager in a small New England business.

Physical examination in February 1975 revealed absent pulses below the left femoral artery that had a decreased pulse and "bruit" (a type of blood flow murmur). The right femoral and all distal right leg pulses were not detected nor were there any murmurs heard. The abdominal aorta had a "bruit". Hair was absent below the ankles bilaterally—a loss in the last five years.

Initial treadmill walking at 2.0 miles per hour produced Grade 3 right calf pain at three-and-one-half minutes on the first effort, after six-and-one-third minutes (following 10 minutes sitting rest) on the second effort, and at eight minutes on the third round. This was taken as encouraging in that it showed a "warm-up" capability with no chest discomfort. The left calf had only Grade 2 discomfort initially with less than Grade 1 on the third effort. Both feet had a waxy pallor after exercise but the left had a far more rapid return of bright red color compared to the right.

On a separate day, a bicycle ergometric trial with two minutes of 150 kilogram meters per minute power output produced only right gluteal (buttock) discomfort when the pedal was under the instep. Grade 2 right calf pain was produced, however, when the pedal was under the ball of the foot (the metatarsal heads—as is the recommended technique with normal function). Continued instep positioned bicycling at 225 kilogram meters per minute had to be terminated at the second minute because of bilateral gluteal muscle weakness rather than disabling pain.

An arm ergometric evaluation likewise produced limiting fatigue before either chest or ischemic arm pain occurred.

The difficulty with John, and one seen with many such patients, was to get him to walk slowly enough in a shopping mall or other indoor location so that he could "warm-up" without experiencing Grade 3 claudication ("intermittent claudication" is the term applied to the crampy discomfort of exertionally induced skeletal muscle ischemia).

He did eventually persist and by May 1975 had slowly pushed up the speed so that he could walk almost indefinitely at 2.0 miles per hour (on a temperate day) and for six to seven minutes at 3.0 miles per hour, both on the horizontal. The main program took place at least three-times-per-day, and during this time he attempts to amble along at a sufficiently slow pace—increased as tolerance increased—so that no more than Grade 2 discomfort was experienced. This was recommended before meals. A limit of 30 minutes was seldom achieved without painless fatigue causing a halt, but a half hour occasionally was accomplished. Brief walks for two to three minutes were recommended every half hour and no less frequently than every hour when awake.

Aspirin, one 5 grain tablet twice a day, was given in hopes it would impede platelet aggregation and a low saturated fat, low cholesterol diet was prescribed with reduced alcohol, and total caloric intake recommended. He did not stop smoking initially and had negligible weight reduction until he began to see progress. The progress seemed to help his motivation in giving up his indulgences. On particularly foul weather days he used a bicycle exerciser until he found he could last long enough to get scrotal and penile numbness that could not be prevented when the horn of the front of the saddle was tilted sharply downward. It was explained to him that his gluteal muscles were temporarily "stealing" blood from other branches of his pelvic arteries and that no permanent damage would result.

Coincident with his improved leg circulation he had more frequent and improved erectile function at more appropriate times with resumed marital relations. As is often the case, however, this uncovered some mild anginal discomfort when he assumed the man-on-top position. Anginal discomfort was less likely to occur if he lay on his back or side and tried to provide quality and duration rather than intensity in his efforts.

Although aortico-iliac angiography was recommended by our group and others, we have not pressed this because of his obvious improvement and now almost overenthusiastic activity. He has enjoyed ski touring in moderate winter weather and bicycling in the summer along with occasional once a week swimming, all of which usually are without chest discomfort. Bicycling can be done with the ball of the foot, and the thigh, hip, and scrotum usually become numb or weak before calf claudication sets in.

Coronary angiograms are contemplated but more to eliminate concern over possible left main stem or equivalent lesions than because his 5-MET exertional limit imposes difficulties in his present life-style. We have not encouraged his jogging and still encourage him to wear steel tipped shoes to protect his toes. If he tolerates more vigorous ski touring this winter, jogging and a return to tennis might be tried. He is walking more and riding the cart less in his resumed golfing activities.

This case illustrates the almost predictable improvement found in most peripheral arterial insufficiency patients if they work at their program intelligently and with persistence. An expensive supervised outpatient program is not usually necessary, but many phone calls and monthly treadmill or bicycle evaluation sessions do much to support motivation and permit adjustments. Peripheral vasodilator medication has not appeared to be particularly useful but hypertensive therapy often appears to be indicated. Beta blockers, however, may permit excessive alpha induced distal vasoconstriction leading to colder hands and feet.

INDEX

349